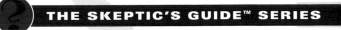

THE SKEPTIC'S GUIDE™ SERIES

Responding to HIV/AIDS

DALE HANSON BOURKE

FOREWORD BY KAY WARREN

TOUGH QUESTIONS, DIRECT ANSWERS

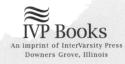

IVP Books
An imprint of InterVarsity Press
Downers Grove, Illinois

InterVarsity Press
P.O. Box 1400, Downers Grove, IL 60515-1426
World Wide Web: www.ivpress.com
E-mail: email@ivpress.com

InterVarsity Press® is the book-publishing division of InterVarsity Christian Fellowship/USA®, a movement of students and faculty active on campus at hundreds of universities, colleges and schools of nursing in the United States of America, and a member movement of the International Fellowship of Evangelical Students. For information about local and regional activities, write Public Relations Dept., InterVarsity Christian Fellowship/USA, 6400 Schroeder Rd., P.O. Box 7895, Madison, WI 53707-7895, or visit the IVCF website at <www.intervarsity.org>.

Scripture quotations, unless otherwise noted, are from the New Revised Standard Version of the Bible, copyright 1989 by the Division of Christian Education of the National Council of the Churches of Christ in the USA. Used by permission. All rights reserved.

While all stories in this book are true, some names and identifying information in this book have been changed to protect the privacy of the individuals involved.

Cover design: Cindy Kiple
Interior design: Beth Hagenberg

ISBN 978-0-8308-3761-8 (print)
ISBN 978-0-8308-6456-0 (digital)

Printed in the United States of America ∞

Library of Congress Cataloging-in-Publication Data

Bourke, Dale Hanson.
  Responding to HIV/AIDS : tough questions, direct answers / Dale Hanson Bourke.
    pages cm. — (The skeptic's guide series)
  Includes bibliographical references.
  ISBN 978-0-8308-3761-8 (pbk. : alk. paper)
  1. AIDS (Disease)—Miscellanea. 2. AIDS (Disease)—Religious aspects—Christianity. I. Title.
  RC606.63.B68 2012
  616.97'92—dc23

                                                              2012045948

P	18	17	16	15	14	13	12	11	10	9	8	7	6	5	4	3	2	1
Y	28	27	26	25	24	23	22	21	20	19	18	17	16	15	14	13		

Contents

How much do you know about HIV/AIDS?

Test your knowledge with these true/false statements (answers on following page).

1. HIV/AIDS can be cured by new drug treatments.   **T   F**

2. In Russia, HIV infections are mostly spread by sexual activity.   **T   F**

3. There are different strains of HIV, some more virulent than others.   **T   F**

4. Sub-Saharan Africa has so many cases of HIV/AIDS because of the large population.   **T   F**

5. India has more people living with HIV/AIDS than any other country in the world.   **T   F**

6. More men than women are infected with HIV/AIDS worldwide.   **T   F**

7. Pregnant women who are HIV positive almost always have babies who are infected.   **T   F**

8. More than a million Americans are living with HIV/AIDS.   **T   F**

9. Men who are circumcised are more likely to be infected with HIV and to spread it to others.   **T   F**

10. A person who has AIDS can be granted asylum in the US on grounds of persecution.   **T   F**

Quiz Answers

1. FALSE. There is no cure for HIV/AIDS, but there are treatments. See page 50.

2. FALSE. Russia has a rapidly growing rate of HIV/AIDS infection primarily due to IV drug use. See page 87.

3. TRUE. Researchers believe there are two primary strains with multiple sub-strains, some more virulent than others. See page 28.

4. FALSE. Sub-Saharan Africa is home to about 10 percent of the world's population but two thirds of all people living with HIV. See page 25.

5. FALSE. Figures for the number of people living with HIV in India were initially overestimated and were readjusted in 2008. The 2009 estimate is 2.4 million, still a large number, but a very small percentage of its population (less than .3 percent). See page 15.

6. FALSE. There are about an equal number of men and women infected worldwide, with more women than men infected in Africa. See page 34.

7. FALSE. Mother-to-child-transmission averages 15 to 30 percent with no interventions but in developed countries has been reduced to a very low rate. See page 27.

8. TRUE. At the end of 2010, approximately 1.1 million Americans were living with HIV or AIDS. See page 20.

9. FALSE. Studies indicate that circumcision helps reduce infection and transmission. See page 42.

10. TRUE. Asylum can be granted to individuals who can prove that their HIV/AIDS status is causing them to be persecuted in their country. See page 91.

Have you ever had an epiphany—a sudden and striking revelation in which you understand a problem from a new and different perspective? In the spring of 2002, that's exactly what happened to me. I was sitting in my living room in affluent Orange County, California, sipping a cup of tea and flipping through a news magazine, completely unaware that life as I knew it was about to come to an end. I paused on an article about AIDS in Africa—not because I cared but because, for some reason, I was curious. I had heard of AIDS before, but I'd assumed it wasn't really a big deal. I assumed that only people who lived half a world away from me became infected; I assumed that becoming HIV-positive was always a direct result of sinful behavior. I assumed that it had nothing to do with my comfortable life in suburbia. I was wrong in every way.

From reading a simple magazine article I learned that HIV/AIDS is a very big deal, killing more than thirty million people in thirty years, leaving fifteen million boys and girls orphaned on the continent of Africa. I learned that more than a million of my fellow Americans are also infected. I was stunned and horrified, suddenly aware of my own ignorance, apathy and prejudice. What had started as a relaxing way to spend an hour became the launching point for a new way of life, a new career, a consuming passion: how to end AIDS in my lifetime.

In the ensuing years, there have been awe-inspiring scientific and medical breakthroughs that have turned a diagnosis of HIV or AIDS from a death sentence into a manageable chronic illness. There is realistic hope for the elimination of mother-to-child transmission and no more AIDS-related deaths in the very near future. But this is not the time to relax our determination or pull back our compassion. There is much yet to accomplish, and finally getting to an AIDS-free generation will require not only the best efforts from the fields of research, science, medicine, philanthropy and government, but from the church of Jesus Christ as well.

When God got my attention about HIV/AIDS and invited me to become an advocate, I was completely ignorant about the pandemic. In an urgent search for information, I read every book I could get my hands on, devoured newspaper and magazine articles, went on every website that talked about HIV, and made the acquaintance of physicians, researchers and people living with the virus. I needed to learn about this devastating virus that was wreaking havoc in the lives of millions of men, women and children. Much of what I read was complicated and geared for professionals; there was next to nothing published for average people who wanted to become literate about HIV/AIDS.

I was so grateful, then, when Dale Hanson Bourke's first edition of *The Skeptic's Guide to the Global AIDS Crisis* came across my desk in 2004. Finally, a comprehensive yet simple book that put the basic facts into a format anyone could understand. I bought the book in large quantities to hand out to people in our ministry who were interested in learning more about HIV, and when the revised and expanded version came along two years later, I bought even more books! Now *The Skeptic's Guide* is part of the newcomer's kit we give to all who join the HIV/AIDS Initiative at Saddleback Church. There is no other book written about HIV/AIDS for laypeople that is as complete and helpful as Dale's. Now in its third edition, retitled as *Responding to HIV/AIDS*, it will remain on my "must read" book list!

Kay Warren

Acronyms

AIDS	Acquired Immunodeficiency Syndrome
ART	Antiretroviral Therapy (or Treatment)
ARV	Antiretroviral
CD4	Cluster Designation 4
CDC	The Centers for Disease Control and Prevention
CSW	Commercial Sex Worker
DNA	Deoxyribonucleic Acid
FBO	Faith-based Organization
FDA	Food and Drug Administration
FGM	Female Genital Mutilation
FSW	Female Sex Worker
HAART	Highly Active Antiretroviral Therapy
HIV	Human Immunodeficiency Virus
IAVI	International AIDS Vaccine Initiative
ILO	International Labor Organization
MSM	Men who have Sex with Men
NGO	Non-governmental Organization
NIH	The National Institutes of Health
PEPFAR	President's Emergency Plan for AIDS Relief
PLWHA	People Living With HIV/AIDS
PMTCT	Preventing Mother-to-Child Transmission
RNA	Ribonucleic Acid
STD	Sexually Transmitted Disease
UNAIDS	Joint United Nations Program on HIV/AIDS
UNICEF	United Nations Children's Fund
USAID	US Agency for International Development
WFP	World Food Program
WHO	World Health Organization
WTO	World Trade Organization

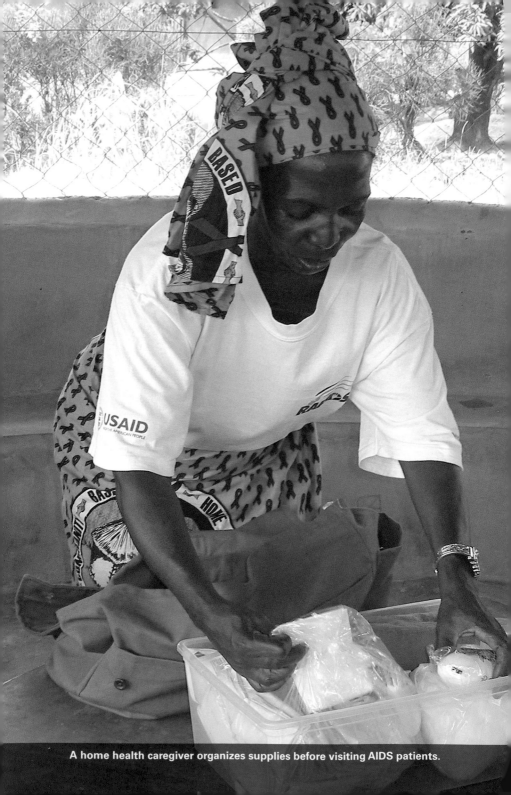

A home health caregiver organizes supplies before visiting AIDS patients.

Introduction

I am not an AIDS expert. Quite the opposite, in fact. I am an ordinary woman who had heard enough about HIV/AIDS to know it was a big problem but not enough to worry about it. I had the good old American belief that if I really needed to know something about HIV/AIDS, I'd get an official notice in the mail, or the newspapers would carry big headlines.

No notice came, and the headlines only confused me. AIDS stories carried incomprehensible statistics and arguments over drugs, treatments, politics and issues I had neither the time nor the inclination to explore. I figured I'd let everyone fight it out and get back to me when they had settled the real issues. After all, if things were so bad, why did everyone waste time bickering?

Like many people, I had become a skeptic about HIV/AIDS. The panic in the United States in the early 1990s had given way to moderation and the understanding that people with HIV/AIDS were not a serious threat to me or my children. Maybe it had just been a passing phase.

Unlike most people, I had the opportunity to travel to Africa and Asia over the course of the last two decades. There I was confronted with the irrefutable evidence that I—like many people—was missing something.

In Africa I saw roadside stands with wooden coffins being sold as quickly as they could be made. In Asia I visited a home for sick and orphaned children whose mothers had died of AIDS. In one country, I met a wrinkled and stooped-over woman who, barely able to walk, had to care for ten children, including an infant. Through a translator, she explained that these were her grandchildren, the survivors of her own sons and daughters, all of whom had died of AIDS. "Pray for me that I will live long enough to raise these children," she implored, her eyes filled with tears.

It didn't take long for these encounters to motivate me to action. But what could I do? It seemed like there was an immense gap between what I knew and what it would take to really help someone.

I looked for a basic book that would help me understand the situation. I found some good material, but most of it raised more questions. As I became more interested in the topic, I began to ask other people what they knew. Soon I realized that when it comes to HIV/AIDS, most of us have a pretty steep learning curve.

This book grows out of the questions I and many others have asked about HIV and AIDS. The answers come from interviews, other books and official statistics provided by the World Health Organization and the United Nations. I try to deliver the most basic facts, explaining medical and political issues in everyday language.

The first edition of this book (*The Skeptic's Guide to the Global AIDS Crisis*) was published in 2004. This revised edition comes at a point in time when there is much to celebrate. In many countries, infection rates have stabilized or even begun to come down. No longer considered a death sentence, HIV is now treated as a chronic disease. Treatment, once costly and not widely available, now reaches almost half of all people infected with HIV in the world. And perhaps most heartening, faith communities, schools, civic groups, nonprofits and even businesses have all become partners in fighting the disease and caring for those affected by it.

Over the past decade I have been honored to meet many men and women who have worked tirelessly to respond to the pandemic. Some have pioneered medical treatments and conducted life-saving research. Others have cared for those who were ill or for children left orphaned by the disease. Still others have provided creative income-generating programs or raised awareness about the disease. Even though no one has found a cure, the response of so many individuals has effectively stopped the disease in its tracks.

The tone at the July 2012 International AIDS Conference in Washington, D.C., was markedly distinct from that of previous conferences. Yes, there was still much work to be done, but more than ever there was hope. Hope for a cure. Hope for universal treatment. Hope for prevention of all mother-to-child transmission.

From the smallest villages in Africa to the largest corporations in the United States, people are responding to a once overwhelming threat with creativity and compassion. My hope is that this very basic book will continue to be a tool to help in those efforts.

From here you can read more books, listen to experts, tell someone else, start a study group or pray. By reading this book, you take a step toward understanding. Just as education is the first step in preventing the spread of HIV/AIDS, so it is also the first step in combating the type of skepticism that spreads complacency.

Dale Hanson Bourke

Alive & Kicking provides soccer balls with health messages made by local people who need jobs.

While interviewing a variety of people from different walks of life, similar questions arose about HIV/AIDS. Following are some of the basic questions and answers. Almost all of these are discussed in more detail later, but if you're looking for a quick overview, this section is for you.

Is HIV/AIDS still an international crisis?

HIV/AIDS is the biggest public health problem the world has ever faced. It has already surpassed the bubonic plague, which wiped out 25 million people—one quarter of Europe's population at the time. Before treatments became widely available, an estimated 3 million people died each year from AIDS. In 2011, there were still 1.7 million HIV/AIDS deaths throughout the world.

HIV/AIDS is found in every country in the world. The highest number of infected people lives in Africa, but countries in Asia also experienced a rapid rate of growth. Because of their large populations, China and India report high numbers of infections, even though those infected account for a small percentage of the population.

HIV/AIDS typically infects people in the prime of life, often depriving children of their parents and communities of their most productive workers. Young people, ages fifteen through twenty-four, now account for 42 percent of new infections.

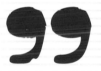

"We are daily standing by while millions of people die for the stupidest reason of all: money."

Bono,
recording artist
and AIDS activist

Since some people are HIV-positive for years without showing symptoms, no one really knows the exact number of infections. Many people in poorer countries are never tested, and many who die of AIDS-related infections are officially listed as succumbing to tuberculosis or malaria.

UNAIDS (see p. 24) estimates that there were 34 million people living with HIV at the end of 2011.

What is the difference between an epidemic and a pandemic?

An epidemic is an illness that occurs and spreads to many more people than would be statistically expected during a point in time. A pandemic is an epidemic that occurs over a large geographic area, usually worldwide.

What do all the initals mean?

HIV stands for Human Immunodeficiency Virus. *Human* means it affects men, women and children. *Immunodeficiency* refers to a decline in the body's natural ability to fight infection. *Virus* means it is a small, infectious organism that reproduces inside a person. AIDS stands for Acquired Immunodeficiency Syndrome. *Acquired* means it is not genetic. *Immunodeficiency,* as with HIV, means that the immune system has become weak or ineffective. *Syndrome* refers to a group of symptoms that occur together and characterize a disease.

Another acronym associated with HIV/AIDS is ART, which stands for Antiretroviral Therapy. ART offers treatment of HIV/AIDS but not a cure. The drugs help a person fight the virus and improve the ability to resist other infections. ART reduces the rate of replication of retroviruses such as HIV. Retroviruses are a particular type of virus that store their genetic information on an RNA molecule instead of a DNA molecule, which is partly why this disease is more difficult to tackle than others.

A more detailed list of acronyms and their meanings appears on page 9.

> *"AIDS is the greatest weapon of mass destruction on earth."*
>
> Colin Powell, Former US Secretary of State

What's the difference between HIV and AIDS?

AIDS and HIV are not the same thing. A person may be infected with HIV for many years before developing AIDS. AIDS is considered to be the last stage of the illness resulting from the HIV virus.

What are the symptoms of HIV?

A person with HIV may not show any major symptoms of infection. There may be flulike symptoms in the first month or two, such as fever, headaches or swollen glands. During this period, the person may not test positive for HIV but is able to transmit the disease.

After the initial phase, a person may be free of symptoms for many years. During this time, however, the virus is invading and attacking a person's CD4 cells—often known as T-cells, the body's primary defense against viruses and bacteria. A healthy person has a T-cell count of 500–1500. A person with a high T-cell count is waging a war on an internal infection. But when HIV begins to take over, T-cells are slowly defeated and destroyed. According to the Centers for Disease Control (CDC), when a person with HIV has a T-cell count at or below 200, or has a related opportunistic infection, the person is considered to have AIDS—the most severe manifestation of HIV.

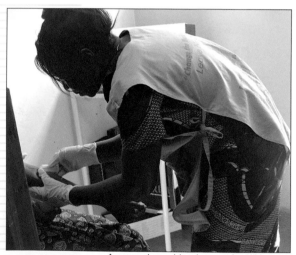

A nurse draws blood to test for HIV and other diseases.

With such a low T-cell count, a person is susceptible to other infections which the body might ordinarily be able to fight. In developing countries, someone with a suppressed immune system can readily contract tuberculosis, malaria, hepatitis or other diseases commonly occurring in the environment. At that point, a person with AIDS can become a carrier of other highly communicable diseases, creating additional health risks for other people.

How are HIV and AIDS diagnosed?

A simple, quick oral test called a "rapid test" can be administered in a clinic, at a doctor's office or by a health practitioner. Unless the infection occurred very recently, if the test is negative, the person is probably not infected. If the test is positive, a blood test is used to determine whether the person is, in fact, HIV-positive. If a person has been exposed to the virus or engaged in risky behavior in the past six months, he or she should be retested.

AIDS can be diagnosed either through measuring the T-cell count or when a number of opportunistic infections or cancers become present in a person with HIV.

FACT:
Each day,
nearly 5,000
people die
due to AIDS.

How are HIV and AIDS treated?

Antiretroviral therapy (ART) has been effective in treating both HIV and AIDS (see p. 50).

Everyone panicked when AIDS was first reported, but now things don't seem so bad. Were we overstating the problem?

99

"Years from now, the AIDS pandemic will be judged as one of those rare crossroads in human history, where everything that comes after it will be seen through its lens."

Richard Stearns, president of World Vision

When the first cases of AIDS were reported in the United States, some of the best medical minds went to work on the problem. The blood supply was tested and purged of potentially infected blood. "At-risk" populations were urged to have HIV tests. The fact that the gay community was hardest hit also meant that a group of people who were generally well-educated and well-resourced brought considerable attention to the problem. With high visibility, most people in the United States quickly learned about AIDS and how it was transmitted.

Although more than 600,000 individuals have died of AIDS in the United States, the rate of infection decreased significantly since the 1980s but has remained fairly steady for the past decade according to the Centers for Disease Control (CDC). The CDC reports nearly 50,000 new infections in the United States each year, and of the approximately 1.1 million people living with HIV, as many as 18 percent do not know it. This has led the CDC to urge all Americans between the ages of thirteen and sixty-four to be routinely screened for HIV as part of their medical exam, and to recommend annual screening at minimum for those in high risk categories.

In poor countries, many people do not know about the risk of HIV and AIDS. When people in impoverished villages are infected, they are often already in bad health and malnourished, so their bodies have difficulty fighting the disease. Inefficient healthcare systems can spread the infection through tainted blood supplies and nonsterile instruments and facilities. Lack of understanding has also led to myths and denial, which has only helped spread the disease. For many years, some governments lacked the will to admit the problem existed, and even when they did, they had limited resources to address it. Some countries still have few testing facilities.

FACT:
Globally, most people living with HIV or at risk for HIV do not have access to prevention, care or treatment.

Wasn't Magic Johnson diagnosed with AIDS but is still fine?

Magic Johnson, the famous basketball player, disclosed in 1991 that he was HIV-positive, though he had not developed AIDS. The virus was discovered at a very early stage, and as an athlete in top condition, Johnson's immune system was probably very strong. He was able to receive the best medical care and was immediately placed on a regimen of drug treatments. (See the discussion of drug treatments on page 50.) Because of this treatment, the HIV virus has remained at a very low level in his system.

Johnson's example illustrates how drug treatments can not only prolong the life of someone who is HIV-positive but can offer the chance for a relatively normal and active life. Now that drug treatments are more widely available and people do not believe that being HIV-positive is a death sentence, they are more likely to get tested.

Why would the US government declare the HIV/AIDS pandemic a threat to national security?

"Please pray that I will live long enough to raise these children."

Malawian woman raising ten grandchildren after her own children all died of AIDS

In 2000, the US government declared the HIV/AIDS pandemic a threat to national security. One reason is that the world is increasingly interconnected. The United States is one day's travel away from many countries.

In addition, in some countries, AIDS has primarily affected the young adult population, leaving only children and the elderly behind. The average age in many African countries, for example, has declined significantly over the last decade. As a consequence, many of these countries have stalled or moved backward in education, healthcare, agriculture and other development indicators. Children in these countries will enter adulthood being closely connected to the United States through travel and communication but having backgrounds of poverty and hardship.

Where did AIDS come from?

AIDS was first clinically identified in 1983, but it is believed to have existed for many years before that. The virus closest to it is simian immunodeficiency virus, a disease found in monkeys in equatorial

Africa. Some believe that the virus jumped from animals to humans when infected "bush meat"—the meat of monkeys—was eaten, a common practice in that region.

Scientists do know that other viruses jump from animals to humans, including some forms of influenza and the disease known as SARS.

Some believe that HIV/AIDS may have existed in Africa for decades before it was clinically identified, providing the virus with the opportunity to mutate and more efficiently infect humans. How it first jumped to humans may never be known, but it probably happened decades ago. For many years in Africa, there was a mysterious disease called "Slims." Infected people tended to lose weight and become very thin. (Some in Africa still use this term to refer to those with HIV infections.)

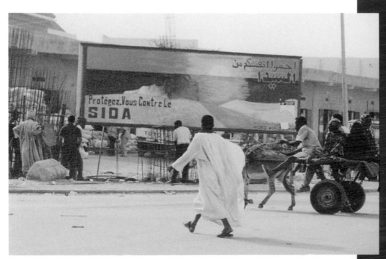

Mauritania was one of the African countries taking a lead in AIDS prevention. This billboard appeared in 1995.

What is UNAIDS?

The United Nations Program on HIV/AIDS (UNAIDS) is a joint program of eleven organizations, including the United Nations Children's Fund (UNICEF); the World Food Program; the United Nations Development Program (UNDP); the International Labor Organization (ILO); the United Nations Population Fund (UNFPA); the World Health Organization (WHO); the United Nations High Commission on Refugees (UNHCR); UNWomen; the United Nations Educational, Scientific and Cultural Organization (UNESCO); the World Bank; and the United Nations Office on Drugs and Crime (UNODC).

FACT:
HIV infections are found in every country in the world.

The purpose of UNAIDS is to lead and inspire the world in achieving universal access to HIV prevention, treatment, care and support. UNAIDS provides the information most often used when talking about the pandemic and plays a central role in coordinating responses. The UNAIDS website, www.unaids.org, is one of the best places for reliable information about AIDS.

What is sub-Saharan Africa, and why is AIDS so bad there?

Sub-Saharan Africa is the part of Africa south of the Sahara Desert. Although this is the largest part of Africa geographically, it tends to be sparsely populated

except in major cities. It is usually considered to include forty-eight countries, many of which are among
the poorest in the world. HIV/AIDS is believed to have
started in this region. This region of Africa is also believed to have the most virulent strain of HIV.

While it is home to only 10 percent of the world's
population, nearly 70 percent of those infected with
HIV/AIDS live in sub-Saharan Africa, according to
UNAIDS. Because of typically poor public health facilities and fragmented communications systems, and because diseases such as malaria, tuberculosis and dys-
entery claimed so many lives for so many years, it is
possible AIDS was not even noticed at first. The biggest
difference between AIDS and the other epidemics in
the region was that AIDS was claiming the lives of
more adults than children.

FACT: Globally, approximately 50 percent of all HIV-positive people are female; in sub-Saharan Africa it averages nearly 60 percent.

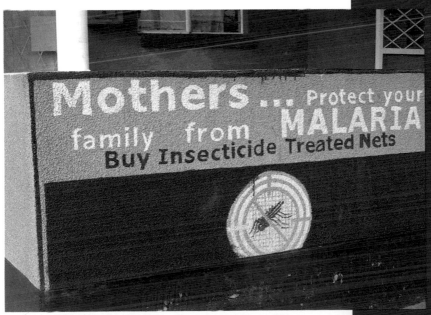

Malaria and HIV/AIDS claim millions of lives in sub-Saharan Africa.

Isn't AIDS mostly a homosexual disease?

FACT:
As of 2009 there were approximately 16.6 million AIDS orphans in the world.

While AIDS in the United States initially had its highest incidence in the gay community, internationally HIV is primarily transmitted through heterosexual sex, intravenous drug use and infection through the blood supply, as well as transmission from infected mothers to their babies. The virus does not exist for long outside of the body, so early fears about contracting the virus through casual contact have been laid to rest. Worldwide, HIV is not primarily a disease of men having sex with men (MSM). More women than men are infected in Africa, and many are infected by their husbands.

HIV is transmitted through contact with blood, semen, vaginal or amniotic fluid, and breast milk. Although the virus is found in saliva, tears and perspiration, the concentration is generally too low for transmission. Unless a person has a cut or tear in the skin, he or she cannot be infected by dealing with human waste of those infected. Neither can a person be infected by sharing utensils with an infected person, swimming or bathing in the same water, being bitten by an insect, or being coughed or sneezed on, according to the Centers for Disease Control (CDC).

Although HIV/AIDS is often a sexually transmitted disease (STD), the risk of transmitting or contracting the disease is increased by the presence of another STD in either partner.

Do infected mothers always pass the virus to their babies?

No. Less than one-third of babies born to women who are HIV-positive are themselves infected. With treatment, transmission to the baby is completely preventable.

Women may pass the virus to their babies in three different ways: during pregnancy through the placenta; during childbirth; and through breast milk. Without treatment, between 15 to 30 percent of babies born to HIV-positive mothers are infected. Caesarian deliveries reduce this to some degree.

One of the earliest stories of hope in the global AIDS crisis was the fact that pregnant women who are HIV-positive can bear children who are free of the virus. Preventing mother-to-child transmission (PMTCT) is an area of great progress in the fight against HIV, since it is now proven that relatively simple drug interventions prevent the infection of an infant whose mother is HIV-positive. In developed countries, such interventions have nearly eliminated mother-to-child transmission. In poor countries, the rate has declined substantially in the last decade.

During the first year, a baby may test positive for HIV because she is still carrying some of the mother's antibodies or because of breastfeeding. This is only because the test measures antibodies, and the child may be HIV-free. A test performed after breastfeeding ends more accurately determines the child's status.

FACT:
Globally, there were 3.4 million children living with HIV in 2010.

Are there different types of HIV?

Yes. Experts believe there are at least two distinct strains of the virus, with many subtypes. The virus appears to be very adaptable and seems to mutate. Certain strains or subtypes seem to dominate in different regions, depending on the primary source of transmission and other factors. Some subtypes cause more rapid progression of the illness.

Why did it take so long to make drugs available to treat AIDS?

Antiretroviral drugs have been widely available in the United States for more than twenty years and have significantly decreased symptoms and prolonged the lives of those who are HIV-positive. Drug therapies have greatly improved over time; treatments known as HAART—highly active antiretroviral therapies— have not only shown marked improvement in suppressing symptoms but have also been shown to suppress the virus itself, making an individual less prone to infect others. This is especially true in reducing transmission from HIV-positive women to their babies.

Drug therapies produced in the United States and Europe were expensive, but the same drugs began to be manufactured much less expensively in other countries. The main cost associated with producing drugs has to do with patents held by drug companies. But the cost of drugs has dropped considerably over the past year, down to less than a dollar a day in many cases.

Treatment with these drugs requires some medical oversight. That makes treatment difficult for many people in developing countries who simply don't have ready access to clinics or doctors. In addition, because there are various strains of the virus, it is important to find the right combination or dosage of drugs to match the nature of the infection. And in order for treatment to be effective, it must continue throughout the lifetime of infected individuals.

FACT: About 40,000 new infections occur each year in the United States.

Why isn't the media reporting more about HIV/AIDS?

HIV/AIDS infection rates are generally reported each year when UNAIDS and the World Health Organization (WHO) issue their annual reports. But otherwise, AIDS is no longer news. Most infections and deaths continue to occur in Africa, and some critics note the dearth of any reporting on Africa. Tuberculosis and malaria have been killing millions of people in African countries for years, but an outbreak of influenza in the United States typically gets far more coverage.

HIV/AIDS is an ongoing crisis that has been around for thirty years. Sadly, most reporting is done only when there is controversy.

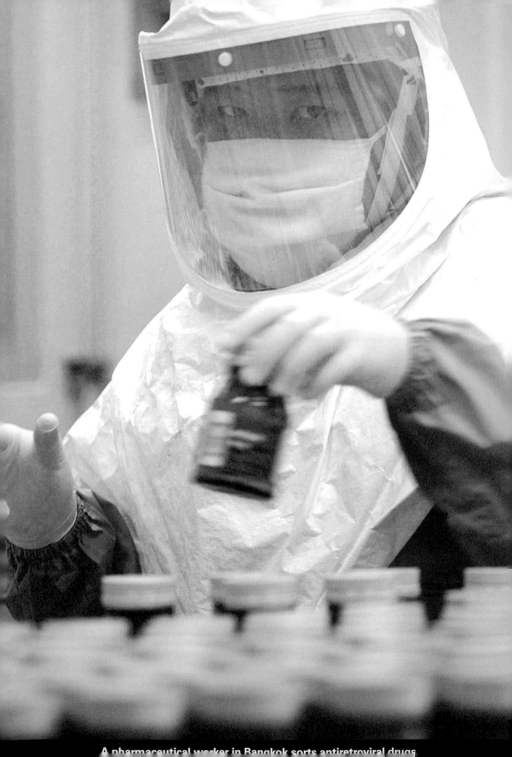

A pharmaceutical worker in Bangkok sorts antiretroviral drugs.

The various medical and public health issues associated with HIV/AIDS are complex and dynamic. These answers offer basic explanations of many questions people have asked about health-related issues.

How was HIV/AIDS discovered?

Evidence of what was later identified as HIV infection was seen in various countries by the late 1970s. Doctors began to see an increasing number of patients with an unusual strain of pneumonia and rare cancers. Some noticed that it appeared most often in gay men and began to call it Gay-Related Immune Deficiency Syndrome, or GRID. In 1983 the human immunodeficiency virus was first isolated by Luc Montagnier at the French Institut Pasteur. It was called lymphadenopathy-associated virus (LAV). Then in the United States Robert Gallo of the National Cancer Institute discovered something he called HTLV-3. At some point the research community realized that Gallo and Montagnier had discovered the same virus, and in 1986 it was renamed HIV.

Because there was a belief that a vaccine would soon be developed, the United States and France disagreed over who had discovered the virus first and who would control the rights to what would presumably be a lucrative patent. Eventually the French researcher was deemed to have discovered the virus. No vaccine has yet been developed.

The statistics about HIV/AIDS seem confusing. Are rates going down?

"Religious leaders are zealous to know more about HIV/ AIDS, and with more information, we'll be able to fight the epidemic more effectively."

Sheikh Ali Banda, Kuomboka Islamic Center, Lusaka, Zambia

Measuring the rate of infection and even death in a pandemic is daunting, but this is especially true with AIDS. The majority of people who are HIV-positive don't even know they are infected. Through lack of understanding or desire to avoid stigma, AIDS deaths are sometimes attributed to tuberculosis or another disease. And of course many of those with immune systems compromised by AIDS actually do succumb to other diseases. In the early days of the pandemic, some countries tried to hide their AIDS problem, fearing that it would hurt tourism or make the country seem vulnerable.

Because of all those factors, numbers relating to AIDS are almost always stated as estimates and in ranges, and various methods are used to continue to refine the numbers. Between 2002 and 2003, the groups involved in developing estimates agreed on more accurate ways to arrive at their figures. The numbers of those infected, released in 2003, appeared to be lower than the previous year, but they were simply a revised, more refined estimate. Further changes were made in 2005 reports to make comparisons among countries more accurate.

For many years the infection rate appeared to be declining. In fact, the rate of deaths was growing faster than the infection rate; people were no longer counted as infected because they had become part of the mortality statistics.

The good news is that with treatment more widely available, the number of AIDS-related deaths is decreasing in most countries. But the number of people living with HIV is increasing, both because people are living longer and because more and more people are getting tested and diagnosed. The rate of new infections is therefore a good measure of the effectiveness of prevention methods, and the death rates are a way to assess the effectiveness of treatment.

FACT: *In 2010, more than 6.6 million people were being treated for HIV.*

Why do some statistics use the "incidence" of HIV/AIDS while others discuss the "prevalence"?

Incidence is used to measure the number of new infections. Annual incidence figures subtract one year's numbers from the previous year's. If you look at the incidence of infections year to year, you can see whether the epidemic is increasing.

Prevalence measures the percentage of the total population infected at a given point in time. When related to HIV/AIDS, prevalence is usually expressed as a percentage. A country with a large population may have many new cases but a small prevalence rate. Conversely, a country with a small population might have the same incidence rate as another country but a much higher prevalence rate.

According to the World Health Organization, in 2009 the countries with the highest *prevalence* rate of

HIV were Swaziland, Botswana, Lesotho, South Africa and Zimbabwe. But South Africa's population is much greater than the other countries, so its *infection* rate, an estimated 5.3 million people, is the largest in the world.

Some researchers believe that when the prevalence rate reaches 5 percent, the infection "takes off" in the total population and begins to increase at a higher rate throughout the country.

How is life expectancy measured?

Life expectancy is the level of mortality in a population at a particular time. It is measured in years and basically gives the average age at which a person in that population could expect to die.

Life expectancy is viewed as a health indicator and is a way to view the overall well-being of a population. Infant mortality rates also affect life-expectancy measures. In many African countries, life expectancy has dropped considerably due to HIV/AIDS because such a large number of people die at relatively early ages.

Is it easier for a woman to be infected through sex than for a man?

Internationally, the rate of infection is about equal between men and women. But according to the World Health Organization (WHO), in Africa women are more likely to be infected than men and now account for 60 percent of infections.

A woman is more likely to be infected by her partner because she is more likely to harbor infected fluids in her body, where they have more opportunity to enter her bloodstream. The practice of female circumcision, also called female genital mutilation (FGM), makes a woman more likely to have complications, including infections, which also make her more vulnerable to HIV.

Sexual violence against women is all too common throughout the world, and in many cultures women are more vulnerable to infection because of their low status in society and in the family—as well as a sexual double standard which exposes them to many risk factors. In some societies a woman is expected to be submissive to her partner; she may not feel entitled or be afraid to suggest the use of condoms, even if she suspects he has had other partners.

Arranged marriages are common in some countries, and age disparity is also common, since the girl's family seeks a husband who is already well established in an occupation, whereas the man is seeking a young girl more likely to be a virgin and uninfected. Girls who are sexually initiated in adolescence are thought to be more vulnerable to tears and abrasions, therefore more susceptible to infections.

In some African countries, there is a belief that having sex with a virgin will cure AIDS. This myth has contributed to an alarming increase in the rape of young women and girls.

Poverty places pressure on girls and women, who often resort to exchanging sex for cash or gifts such as educational fees and even food.

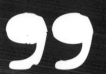

"Any effective initiative to combat the spread of AIDS must . . . eliminate the market for sex trafficking and drastically reduce the instances of rape and other sexual assaults."

Gary Haugen, president, International Justice Mission

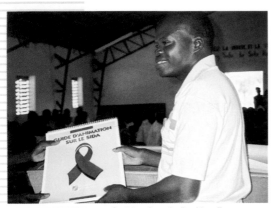

Seminarians in Burkina Faso receive training on AIDS as part of their preparation for ministry.

Sex is still a taboo subject in many countries, and most youth do not receive any kind of sex education in the family or in school. Deeply ingrained gender roles require that girls, especially, are expected to be sexually naive, inexperienced and submissive, while for men multiple partners is a mark of virility.

Speaking to the International AIDS Conference in Bangkok in July 2004, Stephen Lewis, the UN Special Envoy for HIV/AIDS in Africa, called for governments to enact and enforce laws against rape, sexual violence, discrimination, loss of property rights and other situations that hurt women. He also asked for laws to raise the legal marriage age. When he spoke to the same group in 2006, he noted that little progress had been made.

Why are sexually transmitted diseases (STDs) a factor in HIV/AIDS transmission?

Many STDs cause ulcers, sores or other breaks in the skin, which make HIV infection easier to transmit into the bloodstream. In addition, doctors believe that when a person's immune system is already fighting another

STD infection, the very cells the HIV infection are seeking to invade are concentrated and therefore more easily infected in large numbers.

What are people referring to when they talk about the ABCs of AIDS?

When Uganda's President Museveni launched a program to raise awareness and reverse the spread of HIV/AIDS in his country, a major part of the program was education about prevention. In an effort to help spread the message in a simple way, it was promoted as the ABCs, in that order of priority. A is for "abstinence," B is for "be faithful" and C means "use condoms." Another phrase associated with the effort was "Zero Grazing," referring to the practice of keeping cattle within their boundaries and out of neighbors' fields, and applied in this case to encourage fidelity. Other countries adopted the lessons learned from Uganda and the "ABCs of AIDS" became a common way to discuss behavioral change for prevention.

"A whole generation of young people today has never known a world free of HIV/AIDS."

Ann Veneman, former executive director, UNICEF

Why is there so much controversy associated with the ABCs of AIDS?

Edward Green, a Harvard medical anthropologist who studied the "ABCs of AIDS" initiative, observes in his book *Rethinking AIDS Prevention* that since in Ugandan

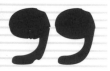

"When a snake comes into the house, we do not stop to ask where the snake came from before we kill the snake."

African saying

culture men often had several sexual partners (a practice widely accepted even by faith leaders), the primary emphasis of the program was on marital faithfulness ("be faithful," or "zero grazing").

According to Green's findings, the use of condoms were weaker factors in prevention in Uganda than monogamy, partner reduction and abstinence. This was due to many reasons, including the fact that condoms were not widely available, especially early in the effort. Moreover, Ugandan men resisted using condoms even when they were available. Meanwhile, partner faithfulness became part of a cultural movement that changed the way Ugandan society viewed sexual experience, especially among young people, increasing the impact on abstinence and faithfulness in sexual relationships.

Green's findings were widely accepted in the United States by faith communities and promoted by the Bush administration. Abstinence became a priority in the prevention goals of the president's AIDS initiative, and approximately 30 percent of US funding was designated for abstinence-based prevention programs. Some faith-based organizations resisted promoting the use of condoms, placing more emphasis on abstinence and fidelity. Thus, abstinence programs became associated with what some considered a conservative agenda.

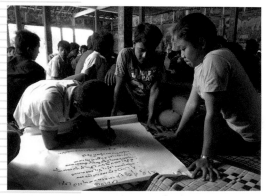

HIV and AIDS education program for young people in a Buddhist temple in Thailand.

Some critics felt that the emphasis on abstinence was unrealistic, especially for women and girls who had little power to resist the advances of men in their culture. Others believed that funding programs that promoted abstinence more than condom use was pushing an American point of view.

Later studies of Uganda showed that condom usage was a significant factor in the decline of infections, and "abstinence only" programs had often proven ineffective. Sadly, the infection rate began to rise again, 6.5 percent in 2009—still less than the initial measure of 18 percent in 1992 but higher than the 4.1 percent achieved in 2003.

Since that time, most prevention programs have emphasized a combination of methods to improve effectiveness.

> **99**
>
> *"[I pledge] to protect myself and to protect others under all circumstances from catching or passing on the AIDS virus."*
>
> Africa 2015 Pledge

What are microbicides?

Microbicides are usually gels or foams that can be used to destroy bacteria or viruses. Because it has been difficult to get men in many cultures to use condoms consistently, attention is being placed on finding ways for women to protect themselves, especially by using something that is not obvious to their partner. A number of clinical studies have been conducted in recent years, but there is still no microbicide that is effective enough to be used in HIV prevention.

Why do some groups oppose the use of condoms?

There are organizations that do not promote the use of condoms at all, while other groups simply promote certain types of prevention more than condom usage. Some religious organizations believe that condom use encourages promiscuity or early sexual activity. Others oppose all methods of birth control, including condoms. Some feel that condoms are undependable and should not be encouraged over abstinence. Others point out that the cost of condoms is too great of a burden on the poor, and it is not realistic to believe they will be used regularly.

Do condoms stop the transmission of sexually transmitted diseases?

Condoms made of natural materials, as opposed to latex or polyurethane, may have pores that allow transmission of microbes associated with STDs. But according to the Centers for Disease Control (CDC) latex or polyurethane condoms, when used correctly and continuously, do prevent the transmission of HIV and other STDs.

Condoms may be reduced in efficacy by heat, sunlight, ozone, lubricants, tears and improper usage. Many men believe condoms reduce sexual pleasure and so prefer not to use condoms. Some women in developing countries don't like condoms because they block their ability to become pregnant. Condoms are expensive for poor people and must be resupplied, although many programs now make them available for free.

Does circumcision prevent HIV infection and transmission?

A circumcised man can be infected with and pass on HIV. But where all other factors are the same, men who are not circumcised have a higher rate of infection and transmission than circumcised men. In recent studies, men who were circumcised were approximately 60 percent less likely to contract the disease.

This difference was first noted in some countries in Africa, where Muslim men are circumcised but Christian men are often not. In the same country, Muslim men often had a lower infection rate. Adult circumcision is now available in most high-incidence countries, and infant circumcision is also being offered in some countries.

The reason for the higher incidence among uncircumcised men, according to the CDC, is that immune cells found in the foreskin (called Langerhans cells) are more susceptible to HIV infection. Uncircumcised men may also have more potential for tearing, providing a way for infection to enter the blood stream.

> "In the context of the fight against HIV and AIDS, I should announce my intention to revive the practice of circumcision amongst young men."
>
> Zulu King Goodwill Zwelithini

Should all baby boys be circumcised?

> "This virus
> is uncanny
> in its ability
> to be able to
> integrate it-
> self into a
> cell, as a
> reservoir,
> and no
> matter what
> we've done
> so far, we
> have not
> been able
> to eliminate
> that
> reservoir."
>
> Dr. Anthony
> Fauci,
> National
> Institutes
> Health

Public health workers endorse circumcision but recognize that encouraging it in poor countries means exposing babies to a procedure often performed in less-than-sterile conditions, increasing the potential for other infection. A number of methods of infant circumcision are being tested that can limit the potential for complications.

In addition, the messages surrounding the procedure must be carefully worded. Circumcision may lower the risk but cannot prevent HIV infections, so men should still use condoms or remain faithful to one partner. And a man who is HIV-positive and has been circumcised may, depending on his viral load, be just as likely to transmit the virus. So it would be a mistake to encourage the belief that a circumcised man is truly a safer sexual partner.

In the United States, approximately two-thirds of all male babies are circumcised. In 1999, the American Academy of Pediatrics changed from recommending circumcision for health reasons to adopting a neutral stance. However, in 2012 the Academy endorsed new guidelines that say the health benefits of infant circumcision outweigh the risks. At this time the general view in the United States is that the decision to circumcise or not should be based on a family's cultural, religious and ethnic traditions, in addition to medical factors. A 2009 CDC report showed evidence that the infant circumcision rate in the United States was declining.

What is female circumcision?

What is sometimes called female circumcision is more widely known as female genital mutilation (FGM) and is condemned by both the World Health Organization and human rights groups. Those who practice it sometimes consider it a coming of age ritual, although it is practiced on girls as young as infants and seems to be most prevalent among girls between the ages of four and eight.

FGM removes part of the female genitalia and is often performed with an unsterilized knife. Besides being painful, the practice often leaves young women with chronic infection problems in both their urinary and reproductive tracts. It can result in incontinence as well as complications in childbirth. The practice itself, as well as the complications associated with it, are considered to further expose girls to HIV infection.

FGM is primarily practiced in certain African countries. It is practiced by members of all religions, although no religion officially requires it, according to the WHO.

> **FACT:**
> *Sexually transmitted infections increase the risk of HIV transmission by at least two to five times.*

Is homosexuality a factor worldwide in HIV/AIDS?

Worldwide, UNAIDS estimates that HIV infections from men to men account for 5–10 percent of all infections, as compared to 61 percent of new infections in the United States, according to the CDC. Homo-

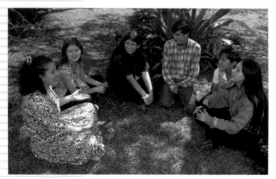

An NGO-led HIV and AIDS information session among young people in Costa Rica.

sexuality does exist in other parts of the world, but men having sex with men (MSM) is highly stigmatized in Africa, Asia and Latin America, and is illegal in many countries.[1] Because relationships between men are far more hidden in developing countries, it is particularly difficult to find effective ways to teach AIDS prevention to men in this group.

Why don't more people get tested?

Until fairly recently, testing could be costly and take a long period of time for results. When withdrawing blood was the only option, medical personnel were needed to conduct the testing. There have been few testing facilities in many poor countries, although that is changing now that oral tests are more accurate and widely available.

Asking to be tested can imply that you have engaged in risky behavior or suspect your spouse. In small communities, this can lead to stigmatizing, whatever the test results. There was also a belief that most people would not want to be tested if there was no cure or treatment. Now that ART is more widely available, people are more willing to be tested.

Does the United States have a policy about HIV testing?

The CDC has issued guidelines for HIV screening in the United States, although not every state has implemented them and not every doctor is following the procedures. Under the new guidelines, there should be routine screening of patients ages thirteen to sixty-four who come in for physicals or other medical procedures. If blood is drawn, the sample could be tested for the presence of HIV. Otherwise a patient could choose an oral test in which gums are swabbed and then tested for HIV antibodies. Anyone who is part of a risk group, including those having unprotected sex or IV drug users, are encouraged to be tested more often.

The reasons for these guidelines include the fact that as many as 18 percent of those who are HIV-positive in the United States do not know they are infected. The CDC estimates that as many as 250,000 people may be unknowingly passing on HIV to their partners. In addition, detecting HIV early allows doctors to begin effective treatments before a person has developed symptoms. And by making testing

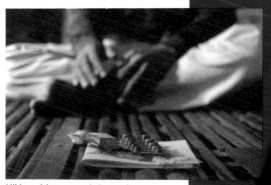

HIV-positive man sitting at home before taking his antiretroviral medicines (ARVs), Cambodia.

routine, just as it is for many chronic but treatable diseases, the stigma is taken away from the disease.

HIV testing is not mandatory in the United States; anyone has the right to ask to be excluded. All pregnant women are urged to have this test, however, since it is possible to prevent transmission to the baby if the mother is HIV-positive.

What are the World Health Organization guidelines for HIV testing?

"The previous generation fought for treatment. Our generation must fight for ⸱ cure."

⸱hel Sidibe,
⸱utive
⸱or,
⸱S

UNAIDS and the World Health Organization (WHO) have developed a policy intended to encourage HIV testing, especially in countries with a high incidence of HIV. The policy can be summarized as the "Three Cs": testing must be *confidential*, accompanied by *counseling* and conducted with informed *consent*.

While UNAIDS/WHO support mandatory screening of blood or organ donors, and of the blood itself, they do not support mandatory testing at public health facilities. They believe that voluntary counseling and testing (VCT) are more likely to result in behavior change.

However, due to the fact that testing is so important, the WHO recently suggested that

> in generalized HIV epidemics, HIV testing and counseling should be recommended to all patients attending all health facilities, whether or not the patient has symptoms of HIV disease and regardless of the patient's reason for attending the health facility. In concentrated and low-level HIV epidemics, depending on the epidemiological and

social context, countries should consider recommending HIV testing and counseling to all patients in selected health facilities (e.g. antenatal, tuberculosis, sexual health and health services for most-at-risk populations). The guidance also includes special considerations for HIV testing and counseling for adolescents and children.[2]

What are the symptoms of HIV infection?

A person who has been infected with HIV may experience swollen glands, fever, nausea, fatigue and overall aches. These symptoms are often mistaken for the "flu" and will eventually subside. After that a person may have no symptoms for years and appear very healthy, even though he or she is infectious. When a person develops AIDS, there is typically weight loss, sores and rashes, lack of energy, fever, swollen glands, chronic diarrhea and such opportunistic infections as thrush.

How close are scientists to finding an HIV vaccine?

Some of the best scientific minds are working on developing a vaccine, but most admit it is extremely difficult. Scientists have begun to look at both the possi-

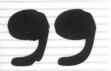

"When there's conflict, drought, famine, major population movement, major military movement, you can suspect that HIV/AIDS is running wild."

Kristin Kalla, former director, CORE Initiative

bility of curing the disease and the greater probability of reducing the viral load of a person who is HIV-positive to an extremely low level. Recent studies show that a person who receives antiretroviral drugs before exposure can reduce the possibility of infection by as much as 96 percent.

The nature of the virus itself makes it hard to attack without killing healthy cells. HIV attaches to the genetic makeup of the cells themselves and masquerades as healthy cell structure. HIV is also a highly adaptive virus, changing forms not only within populations but also mutating within individuals. Finding financing for vaccine research is also difficult, since development of a vaccine can take enormous resources but is extremely risky in terms of payoff.

Scientists also note that immunizations typically rely on injecting individuals with a "watered down" version of a disease so that a person basically gets a mild form of it and then develops immunities to it. Such vaccines are usually developed by studying individuals who have survived the infection and whose bodies have developed natural immunities. While individuals with HIV can greatly reduce the rate of infection through the use of antiretroviral drugs, no one has been found to be virus-free once they have contracted the disease.

In 1996 an international nonprofit organization, the International AIDS Vaccine Initiative (IAVI), was founded in order to increase attention to the search for a vaccine as well as to coordinate efforts in research. IAVI tracks the work of teams doing research in several countries, allowing scientists to try different approaches to finding a vaccine so that no one course is taken exclusively. It also encourages the sharing of information among researchers and helps teams of scientists progress through clinical trials. IAVI insists that any vaccine developed with its support be made available in developing countries at reasonable prices, rapidly and in sufficient quantity. This removes some of the profit incentive that normally spurs drug research but also guarantees that any vaccine that is developed would go to where the need is greatest.

Some who have studied HIV warn that its adaptive nature could make it drug-resistant to any vaccine within a relatively short time frame. This would mean an individual who had been immunized could still be infected by a mutated version of the disease. This might lead to even greater problems, such as people taking fewer precautions, or strains developing that would not respond to treatments. And be-

FACT: *Sub-Saharan Africa is home to 12 percent of the world's population and more than two-thirds of all people living with HIV.*

Estimated AIDS Deaths, 2010

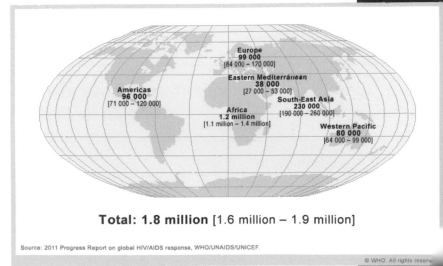

Total: 1.8 million [1.6 million – 1.9 million]

Source: 2011 Progress Report on global HIV/AIDS response, WHO/UNAIDS/UNICEF.

cause of the different strains of the virus, it is possible that a vaccine might be developed that would be effective on one strain but not others.

Public health officials point out that even if an effective vaccine were discovered soon, it would take a massive effort to produce the vaccine and immunize populations.

How are people treated before exposure to HIV?

In couples where one of the partners is HIV-positive and the other is not (called discordant couples) the infection-free partner is given ART called pre-exposure prophylaxis (PrEP). This therapy has been shown to be highly effective in preventing infection. Both partners must remain on the drug treatment regimen to be effective.

Are there different types of drugs to treat HIV/AIDS?

Drugs to treat HIV/AIDS are considered antiretroviral therapy (ART) and act by stopping the HIV from reproducing inside the body, thereby giving the immune system a chance to fight back. There are five main types of ARTs. They are often given in a combination.

Nucleoside reverse transcriptase inhibitors (known

as "nukes") mimic the process the virus uses to invade the cells and then stop replications of the HIV. Two of the more common ARTs, ZT and 3TC, are nukes. Two nukes are sometimes used in combination with a "non-nuke" to prevent mother-to-child transmission.

The second group, non-nucleoside reverse transcriptase inhibitors (known as "non-nukes"), work by blocking a part of the enzyme necessary to produce the viral DNA.

The third group, protease inhibitors (PIs), disable protease, a protein HIV needs to make copies of itself.

Entry or fusion inhibitors block HIV's entry into CD4 cells (see p. 52).

Integrase inhibitors disable integrase, a protein that HIV uses to insert its genetic material into CD4 cells.

Antiretroviral Therapies

Nucleoside reverse transcriptase inhibitors	"Nukes"	Mimic HIV's process, then stop HIV replication
Non-nucleoside reverse transcriptase inhibitors	"Non-nukes"	Block part of an enzyme that produces viral DNA
Protease inhibitors	"PIs"	Disable protease, a protein HIV needs to make copies
Entry or fusion inhibitors		Block HIV's entry into CD4 cells
Integrase inhibitors		Disable integrase, a protein HIV uses to insert genetic material into CD4 cells

A cocktail of three or more drugs is known as highly active antiretroviral therapy (HAART) and is often used with people who have developed AIDS.

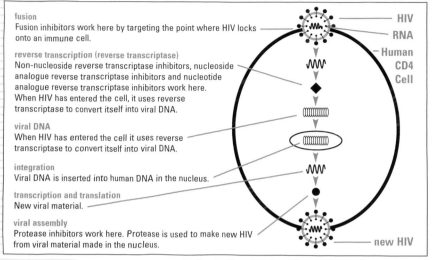

fusion
Fusion inhibitors work here by targeting the point where HIV locks
onto an immune cell.

reverse transcription (reverse transcriptase)
Non-nucleoside reverse transcriptase inhibitors, nucleoside
analogue reverse transcriptase inhibitors and nucleotide
analogue reverse transcriptase inhibitors work here.
When HIV has entered the cell, it uses reverse
transcriptase to convert itself into viral DNA.

viral DNA
When HIV has entered the cell it uses reverse
transcriptase to convert itself into viral DNA.

integration
Viral DNA is inserted into human DNA in the nucleus.

transcription and translation
New viral material.

viral assembly
Protease inhibitors work here. Protease is used to make new HIV
from viral material made in the nucleus.

HIV
RNA
Human
CD4
Cell

new HIV

An illustration showing where antiretrovirals block HIV.

What is meant by retrovirus and lentivirus?

HIV is both a retrovirus and a lentivirus. A retrovirus stores its genetic information on a single-stranded RNA molecule instead of the double-stranded DNA, which is more common among viruses. After a retrovirus penetrates a cell, it uses a special enzyme called a reverse transcriptase to construct a DNA version of its genes, which then is incorporated into the cell's own genetic material.

A lentivirus produces a chronic disease in its host and can remain latent for long periods of time. The time between infection and symptoms can lag by months or years. A lentivirus is a type of retrovirus.

If a person thinks he or she has been exposed to HIV/AIDS, is there anything that can be done?

A treatment known as post-exposure prophylaxis (PEP) can be administered to a person who has been exposed to HIV accidentally, such as a health-worker being pricked by a needle containing infected blood. Post-exposure prophylaxis is started immediately after someone is exposed and consists of antiretroviral drugs that help a person's immune system provide protection against the virus and prevent HIV from becoming established in someone's body. It usually consists of a monthlong course of two or three different types of the antiretroviral drugs that are also prescribed as treatment for people living with HIV.

FACT:
In Russia, heroin is often cheaper than alcohol and is one of the primary reasons, due to shared needles, that HIV infections have risen dramatically there.

How often does sexual contact with an infected person result in transmission?

The infection rate varies depending on the method of transmission, although a person can be infected by only one contact. Male-to-male sexual relations (MSM) tend to transmit the virus more efficiently than male to female. An infected man is nearly twice as likely to infect a female partner as an infected woman is to infect a male partner. Sharing of infected needles almost always leads to new infection, and since the virus enters the bloodstream immediately, the newly infected person may pass on the virus sexually before he or she has any symptoms. When drug use is the primary method of infection, the virus often spreads through the rest of the population rapidly, through shared needles or sexual contact.

What are the side effects of drug treatments for HIV/AIDS?

Side effects vary by drug and individual but may include nausea, headache, diarrhea, fatigue, rashes or fever. It is critical to monitor the side effects in order to adjust dosage or determine if a different drug would be more effective. Also, anti-retroviral drugs (ARVs) may interact with other prescriptions or some herbal treatments. After a period of time, the virus may become resistant to certain drugs, causing patients to change to alternative drug therapies.

Are people in poor countries able to be treated effectively?

Antiretroviral drugs do need some supervision to be administered properly, but they do not need as high a level of care as was once thought. Early courses of ARV treatments were complex, especially those taken in combinations. Now some drugs are combined into a single pill that can in some cases be taken once a day. It is important for a person seeking treatment to be tested accurately and for the treatment to be monitored enough to know whether the drug therapy is working. Side effects must also be monitored.

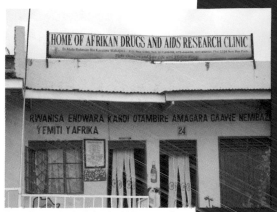

Storefront AIDS clinics in Africa promise natural cures.

For those living in resource-poor countries, the greatest challenges to treatment are often the availability of clean water for taking pills and the adequacy of their diet so that the drugs are not taken on an empty stomach. People whose diets are very poor often have a difficult time staying on the drugs because of stomach upset.

Why can't drugs be made available to all pregnant women who are at risk?

Some doctors suggest that every pregnant woman in highly infected countries receive at least a single dosage of an antiretroviral drug to help reduce the transmission rate to infants. Some ethicists question whether a woman would be provided with enough drugs to prevent transmission to a baby but not enough to prolong her life so she could care for her child.

With a lack of resources to provide drugs to all pregnant women and their babies, most ethicists agree that priority should be given to saving lives.

What is viral load?

The viral load measures the amount of HIV in the blood of someone who is infected. This is an important measure to determine the type of treatment that is indicated, as well as to measure how effective the treatment is. During the course of therapy, a person's viral load should drop to a very low point—almost undetectable by the standard blood test. This does not mean a person is cured; it simply means that the treatment is keeping the virus under control.

What is the "Lazarus Effect"?

A person who has been suffering from HIV or AIDS without treatment may be losing weight and wasting away physically. After a short time on ART, the person begins to gain weight and resist other infections; they literally look as if they have come back to life. In essence, the person appeared to rise from his or her death bed. This dramatic response to treatment, especially for those with very visible signs of AIDS, helped make ARVs popular.

Is the US blood supply really safe?

The Red Cross goes to great lengths to ensure that its blood supply is free of hepatitis, HIV and other diseases. The pre-screening process for potential donors is far more extensive than in the past and disqualifies people who have visited countries with high rates of HIV infection, even people who lived in Europe for more than six months during certain periods of time.

Every blood donation is tested using highly sensitive techniques that are able to detect viruses at a very early point in development. The US blood supply is considered to be completely safe, although all the additional screening has created an ongoing shortage of blood. Because of this, some doctors recommend "banking" blood before an operation. This practice is intended to ensure availability moreso than safety.

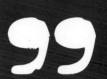

"The number of new infections must be dramatically reduced in the next few years to ensure that antiretroviral treatment remains economically and socially sustainable."

Intensifying HIV Prevention, UNAIDS Policy Paper

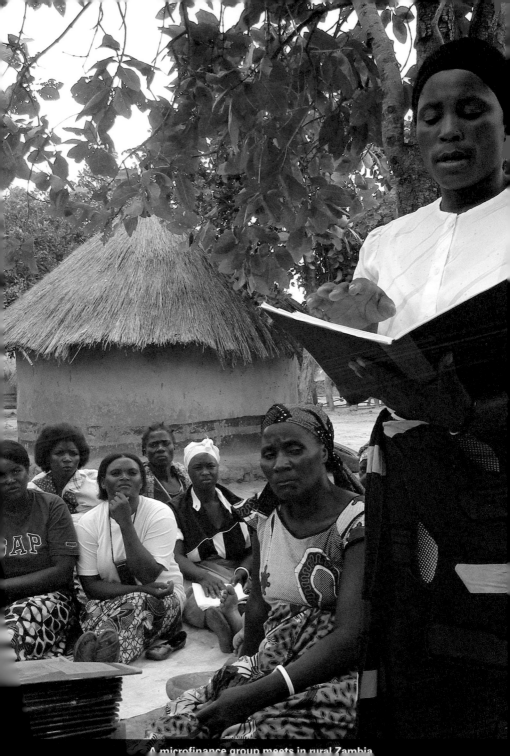

A microfinance group meets in rural Zambia.

Many discussions about AIDS include talk about money. Here are some of the questions people have about the economics of AIDS.

How does the HIV/AIDS situation in other parts of the world affect the US economy?

Most economists believe that in today's global economy, every nation's economic health impacts the others. The global AIDS crisis has devastated many economies in poor and developing countries. This means that those countries are more vulnerable to famines, wars, political instability and declining standards of living.

The CIA has identified the AIDS crisis as a threat to national security because of its destabilizing effects on economies and governments, and because it helps widen the gap between relatively wealthy and poor nations. Since HIV infections are still growing in nations with economic clout and even nuclear weapons, there is a perception that it is in the long-term political and economic interests of the United States to be on the forefront of AIDS treatment and prevention.

It is far more economically beneficial to prevent HIV infections than to treat people with AIDS or to deal with the consequences of widespread illness and mortality.

What are the "next wave" countries?

In 2002 the National Intelligence Council identified China, India, Russia, Ethiopia and Nigeria as the "next wave" countries in the HIV/AIDS pandemic. All had significant and growing infection rates, large populations and governments that had not given fighting the disease a high priority. These countries account for nearly 40 percent of the world's population.

Although these countries represented a later outbreak of the pandemic, by 2007 significant deaths were being reported, and the governments began to take aggressive action. In 2008 China reported 7,000 deaths from HIV in the first nine months of the year, the highest mortality rate for any disease.[3] China's program to test, treat and prevent HIV infections is now a significant part of the country's health program.

Why does AIDS hit economies so hard?

Most people affected by HIV/AIDS are in the prime of life. They are the most productive workers, are earning the most wages and have young children to provide for. They are the backbone of the economies of most countries.

In most developing countries, farming is the primary livelihood, accounting for 70 percent of Africa's employment. Agriculture is labor-intensive and not only provides wages for workers but also produces food for their families. If a worker is ill, there is often no one to take his place, so the ground lies fallow. If a crop isn't planted on time, a family or an entire village may miss the harvest. The food from that harvest may have been intended to supply a year's worth of food for the family or even the whole village.

The World Bank is tracking the impact of HIV/AIDS in other sectors of the economy as well, and has found significant costs associated with absenteeism, lower productivity, employee turnover, increased training and recruitment costs. A severe shortage of teachers and health workers in many countries is attributed to the AIDS crisis.

When adults fall ill or die, their children are taken in by family members and others, meaning fewer adults to work and more children to care for. Often the caretakers are older people who are no longer able to be very productive. Sometimes young people will leave the village to seek jobs in the city. But too often those young people end up in low-paying jobs or are forced into prostitution.

Are the costs of these problems actually measured?

Like most statistics associated with AIDS, figures are approximates, but there are measurements done by such groups as the World Bank, the Food and Agriculture Organization (FAO) and the International Labor Organization (ILO). The ILO works to ensure the human rights of those living with HIV, to help reduce infections in the workplace and to help workers who are living with HIV be more productive.

Other ways to measure the impact include the rising number of children in the labor force, the decline in savings levels, and the sale of family assets in order to care for sick family members or pay funeral expenses.

What are some of the other effects on families and individuals in developing countries?

Having someone in the family who is ill often makes a situation that is already difficult catastrophic. If the person is the primary wage earner, the family can lose all their income and their primary source of food. Children often must stop going to school because they can no longer pay the school fees. Other results include a high risk of sexual and labor exploitation of women and children who are desperate for basic necessities. When a member of the family dies, funeral costs can put the family into debt. Illness and death associated with HIV/AIDS causes a downward spiral for a family, not only reducing their current income and standard of living but also robbing their future chances of moving out of poverty.

What is "transactional sex"?

Transactional sex refers to anytime sex is exchanged for something of value, including money, food or shelter. It refers to everything from formal prostitution to the relationship some young women have with older men in poor countries in which their education is paid for as long as they maintain a sexual relationship with the man.

What is "survival sex"?

This term is somewhat controversial but is used by some to mean either commercial or occasional sexual activity engaged in out of economic desperation. Some organizations and individuals use "survival sex" to distinguish individuals who engage in such activities as a last resort from those who make the choice to be sex workers.

Because of the desperate poverty in many countries and the fact that women often have few or no rights, some are either forced or coerced into sexual relations in order to feed themselves or their children. Children who are orphaned and end up living on the streets sometimes survive by offering sex to adults in exchange for money, food or shelter.

How does labor migration contribute to the pandemic?

In poor areas of the world, it is common for people to move where labor is needed. Sometimes people become migrant farm workers. In Africa, large numbers of people were brought from rural areas to provide inexpensive and plentiful labor for mining.

Because migrant workers are typically men and are away from their families for long periods of time, it is common for prostitutes to congregate in areas where migrant workers live. When the men go home, they may bring with them STDs, including HIV. Based on patterns of infection, it seems clear that the rate of HIV infection follows paths of migrant workers.

People Living with HIV, 2010

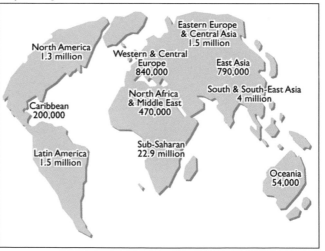

"*My father gave me to a man who promised to feed my family. If I refused to have sex with the man, my family would have starved.*"

Teenage girl in Mozambique

Labor migration is found wherever poverty exists. It almost always breaks down the social and cultural structure and has been responsible for the spread of diseases for decades.

Another pattern of disease runs along African transportation routes. As truckers move across regions, they are often stopped at border crossings and checkpoints for days at a time as they go through immigration and customs formalities. These checkpoints attract prostitutes and petty traders. The pattern seems to indicate that infected truckers spread HIV across a region and among countries.

What is microfinance?
How does it help poor women?

Microfinance is a method whereby poor people are given small loans to help them finance a business. The loans may be as little as $50 and are given to individuals to help them start such businesses as selling vegetables in a market, developing a sewing business, buying tools in order to provide services or purchasing soda for resale. Loans are usually made to people who cannot qualify for commercial loans or who would be charged an exorbitant rate if they did apply for a loan. Many individuals who begin with small loans are able to develop their businesses into enterprises that can provide income for their entire family.

Microfinance is especially helpful for women who have typically relied on their husbands to provide food or income. Some microfinance organizations provide training to young people whose parents are sick or have died so that they can earn a living independently.

Most microfinance organizations are supported by nonprofit groups which help provide the initial capital for the loans. Eventually the loan funds become self-sustaining and may even become commercial banks which provide loans and also accept savings, still dealing primarily with the very poor.

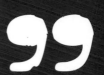

"Nine of every ten people living with HIV will get up today and go to work."

Juan Somavia, International Labor Organization

How does microfinance relate to the AIDS crisis?

Microfinance is typically carried out in small groups, which work together to guarantee each other's loans and provide support during regular meetings. These meetings also provide opportunity for education, especially in the basics of business and health. Because nonprofit organizations typically provide the structure for these groups, they are able to use them as a way to teach AIDS education, especially to women. And because there is a certain amount of group support and pressure, women can learn to stand up for their rights, including asking their husbands to be faithful or use condoms if they suspect them to be HIV infected.

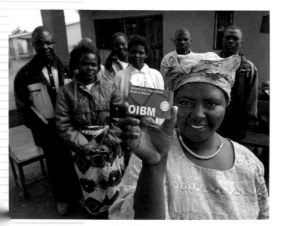

Talekelini Kagaso displays her "smart card" used at the Opportunity Bank of Malawi to prevent her savings from being claimed by relatives or strangers.

Women who have some measure of economic independence are not as likely to succumb to pressure from men to have sex in exchange for food, education or shelter. They are more readily able to find work near their home instead of migrating to cities where they may end up in prostitution.

Microfinance has been so successful in some countries that it has had an impact on the overall economy of the nation. It has helped spur growth outside of cities and has been especially helpful in providing a means whereby women caring for many children can earn an income while staying close to home.

Microinsurance plans are also now available and help pay for unexpected costs such as funerals.

What does debt forgiveness have to do with AIDS?

Many poor countries have an enormous debt burden created by borrowing over the course of decades. Some of these funds were borrowed by corrupt leaders who used the money to finance their own lifestyles. Other funds were borrowed to fund civic projects, but the interest rates were so high that the burden of the debt became too great. Some believe that money was loaned to these countries at very high rates of interest and without concern about what the debt would do to the countries. It would be a little like a bank offering a loan for a million dollar home to a family earning very little money each year. The chances of default would be great. In order to repay their debts, many countries must rob themselves of badly needed funds to provide for transportation, public health, education and communication. Without this infrastructure, it is difficult to combat AIDS.

Jubilee 2000 was a campaign embraced by many humanitarian organizations, religious groups and some governments to promote debt forgiveness in exchange for guarantees that the money would instead go to alle-

> "If there was ever an innocent in the world, it's a little newborn girl in Africa dying of AIDS."
>
> Wesley K. Stafford, Compassion International

viate poverty. Singer Bono and others led the campaign in 2005 to "Make Poverty History" and urged the G-8 countries to forgive the remaining debt.

Are many charities fighting AIDS?

Many international charities have made AIDS one of their primary causes. No matter what the emphasis of the organization, AIDS has an effect on the people they serve. Many groups have received substantial grants through USAID and other government agencies, as well as from foundations and large donors.

As the international response has matured, charities have begun to specialize in areas such as orphan care, assistance to women, education of children, testing and volunteer support for individuals living with HIV/AIDS.

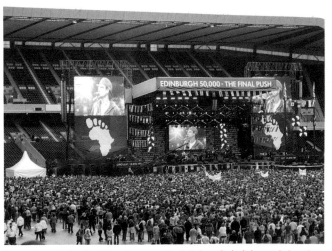

Bono sings at the final Live 8 concert in Edinburgh, helping to bring the attention of the G-8 leaders to AIDS and poverty in Africa.

What is the Global Fund?

The Global Fund for Tuberculosis, AIDS and Malaria (GFTAM, or the Global Fund) was launched in 2002 with the help of the UN and promoted by UN Secretary General Kofi Annan. It was envisioned as an international partnership of public and private interests to help funnel funds directly to countries fighting the three diseases. Because it would offer a coordinated mechanism, the hope was that this one fund would provide an efficient method for funding prevention and treatment at the local level.

Funds have come not only from governments but also from the Gates Foundation, the Rockefeller Foundation and the Clinton Foundation. The fund has a board of directors made up of representatives from governments, the private sector and non-governmental organizations (NGOs), and has a small staff originally seconded from UNAIDS and WHO.

As of 2012, according to the Global Fund's website, the fund has committed $22.6 billion in 150 countries to support large-scale prevention, treatment and care programs against the three diseases.

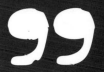

"Valiant, dedicated people . . . know what needs to be done if they can only get the resources they need."

Barbara Wallace, director of HIV/AIDS and health initiatives, CARE

Do we really need to spend more money on AIDS?

According to UNAIDS, an estimated $15.6 billion was spent on HIV and AIDS programs in 2008. But by 2009, the amount had dropped by nearly 10 percent, partially due to the global financial crisis. Many governments are having a difficult time meeting their commitments to fund programs. In addition, there is a movement away from assistance for a single disease; instead, programs are funding total health programs.

Funds are needed for care of orphans, counseling and testing, treatment of those in urgent need of anti-retroviral treatment, and education and prevention.

How much of the money goes to Africa?

Because the highest number of AIDS infections still occur in African countries, Africa continues to receive the majority of funds for treatment as well as prevention. Asia receives the next most funding, followed by Latin America and Eastern Europe.

How can we be sure the money is being used efficiently?

Most programs administered by the UN or through US grants have specific requirements for reporting and meeting goals. Interim reports evaluate progress in meeting the goals; additional funding is not released until specific goals are met. The Global Fund's progress in allocating and monitoring funds is closely scrutinized by the governments, corporations and NGOs that make up the board of directors and provide the funds. Almost all government and large foundation grants have stringent requirements for not only when reports must be filed but what documentation must be included, and progress must be verified by objective parties.

Top Six Government Donors to the Global Fund

Country	Amount Pledged	Amount Given	Period of Pledge
USA	$9.5B	$5.1B	2001-2013
France	$3.8B	$2.4B	2002-2013
UK	$2.2B	$1.4B	2001-2015
Japan	$2.1B	$1.3B	2002-2013
Germany	$2.0B	$1.3B	2002-2013
European Commission*	$1.6B	$1.2B	2001-2013

*The executive body of the European Union, a confederation of 27 member countries located primarily in Europe

Is the United States giving more than anyone else?

According to a report by UNAIDS and the Organization for Economic Development and Cooperation (OECD), the United States is the single largest national donor to worldwide AIDS programs, including the Global Fund. It provides just over half of all funding, followed by the United Kingdom, Japan and the Netherlands.

What types of programs are supported by these funds?

Funding from the Global Fund, as well as PEPFAR and other programs, support HIV/AIDS prevention, testing, treatment and care services, as well as social assistance to those affected by the pandemic.

FACT:
An HIV/AIDS strategy is now part of almost every ministry of health program in the world.

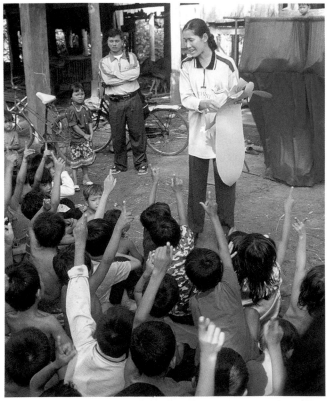

Cambodian children enjoy a puppet show that teaches them about AIDS.

What is the World Trade Organization?

The World Trade Organization (WTO) is the primary body overseeing international trade agreements. It sets trade rules, facilitates trading and negotiates disputes between member countries.

The WTO's main involvement in responding to HIV/AIDS has been in relation to the intellectual property rights of pharmaceutical companies and whether countries can violate patents in order to have access to life-saving generic drugs. Under the Trade-Related Aspects of Intellectual Property Rights Agreement (TRIPS), all countries must comply with patent protection measures involving drugs. However, the Doha Declaration (so named because it came out of a WTO meeting in Doha, Qatar) affirmed that countries may declare a public health emergency and thereby bypass certain patent protections. The Doha Declaration permits countries to legally manufacture or import generic drugs under "compulsory licenses" before patent protections have expired.

FACT:
The acronym for AIDS in French, Spanish and other romance languages is SIDA.

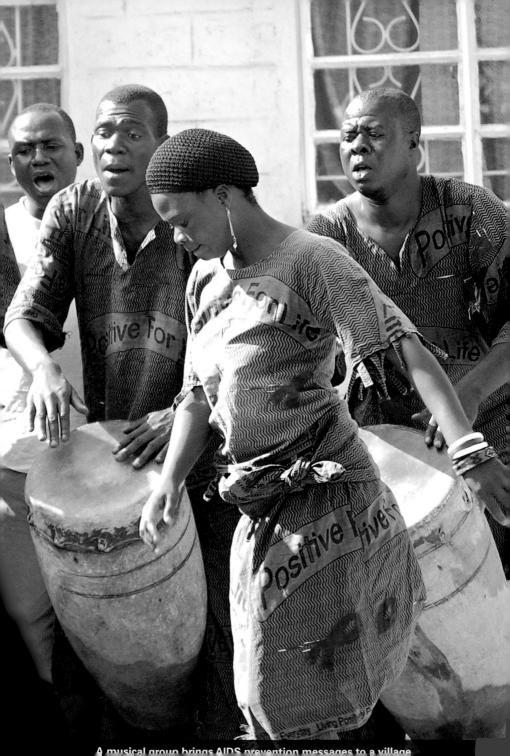

A musical group brings AIDS prevention messages to a village

4. Culture and Practice

We approach any question of culture and belief with our own set of beliefs, norms, prejudices and expectations. Perhaps one of the biggest challenges we all face is recognizing that many of the people affected by HIV/AIDS have neither our experience of the past nor our expectations for the future.

Why are there so many AIDS orphans?

Orphans are described in different ways. There are more than 100 million orphans in the world, using the UN definition (a child under the age of fifteen who has lost one or both parents), but that number includes children who have been orphaned due to wars, disease and other factors. To distinguish just those children orphaned by AIDS can be difficult.

According to the 2011 report of UNAIDS, there are 16.6 million children worldwide who are orphans due to AIDS. The number is so high because HIV-infected people are typically of childbearing age. Women are often infected by their husbands and may find out they are infected only after giving birth to a child who is obviously sick.

Why is there confusion about the number of AIDS orphans?

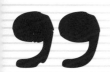

"It is our duty as children of the same God and citizens of the same planet to pool our energies and banish the scourge of AIDS . . . once and for all."

rmer US
sident
linton

Part of the confusion arises because children are not often identified publicly as AIDS orphans since that stigmatizes them and the families who care for them. The current and projected number of orphans, just like all AIDS data, is estimated through statistical models. The modeling techniques have improved over the years, and many experts have now begun to agree on the various assumptions to include in the models. As the methodologies develop and the information on which assumptions are based improves, the numbers change but are increasingly more reliable.

Children may lose one parent to AIDS and continue to live with the other, or they may be abandoned or sent to live with relatives because a parent is too ill to care for them. (Typically, when one parent dies, the other is infected and is ill or dying as well.) If the mother dies and the father is working far away (see p. 63), he may not be able to care for the children. For these reasons, a child who loses one parent to AIDS—whether a father or mother—is considered an orphan.

The vast majority of AIDS orphans live in Africa, where children are traditionally cared for by relatives. This means that families are being strained to deal with the many additional dependents. Sometimes grandparents are caring for their grandchildren after their sons and daughters have died. Increasingly, there are households where the oldest sister or brother cares for the younger children.

Are orphanages the best solution?

African culture has never accepted the concept of orphanages because there is a strong tradition of caring for the children of relatives or friends. But as the cost of caring for so many children proves overwhelming, more child-headed households are springing up. Discussions are taking place about how to care for children in a way that respects tradition but also provides basic care.

There have been some experiments with foster living arrangements, where groups of children are provided and cared for by resident adults who allow them to remain with their closest relatives. This is especially effective in villages where children can remain near their homes and be in a familiar situation.

Institutional childcare has been abandoned in most developed countries because of concerns both about the quality of care and costs. Most experts on childcare worldwide agree that institutional care is much less desirable for the healthy development of children than some kind of family care. Furthermore, it costs much more to care for a child in an institution than in a family, and neither governments nor charities have the necessary funds.

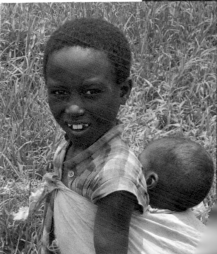

A young girl begs for money to help care for her baby sister in Uganda.

Saddleback Church in California has been a leader in supporting orphan care in Africa through their adoption program, as well as support for local church work with orphans.[4]

Can AIDS orphans be adopted internationally?

Because children carry on traditions, inherit the land, and are keepers of the family name and honor, leaving even distant relatives is very difficult in Africa. What might be considered a "better life" by people in wealthy countries is not always seen as such by poor countries.

Some countries have laws against foreign adoptions, especially by those from overseas. But because of the high number of orphaned children, more countries are quietly relaxing adoption rules.

Is there a crisis in dealing with the elderly in some countries?

In many cultures children are expected to care for their elders. But when so many men and women in their twenties and thirties are dying, their parents have no one to care for them as they age. Since life expectancy is much lower in many developing countries, especially since there may have been little health care and poor nutrition, a person may be considered elderly in his or her fifties.

There are no retirement homes in most countries, nor is there Social Security or pension plans. People who are too old to work or find their own food are totally dependent on younger people. But in many countries, those who are older are caring for their grandchildren and are barely able to cope. Older people who were once revered are now left to fend for themselves.

What is meant by "vulnerable populations"?

In the context of HIV/AIDS, vulnerable populations are defined by UNAIDS as groups that are denied their human rights; have limited access to HIV information, health service and means of prevention; or have limited ability to negotiate safer sex. In most countries this means women and girls, the poor, certain ethnic groups and refugees.

What cultural issues are affected by or affect the spread of HIV/AIDS?

Certain tribal customs in Africa have contributed to the spread of AIDS, especially through families. When a woman's husband dies, she and her children are "inherited" along with his property. According to some traditions, she is expected to become the wife

of one of her late husband's relatives, or to be pu-
rified of her husband's death through sex. This
means that a woman may lose her husband and her
property all at once.

There is also a custom that young women and girls
are to provide sex for an older male relative if he has no
wife. This is seen as a way to thank the relative for providing for the immediate family's needs.

There is a widespread belief that a woman's worth is
primarily related to her ability to bear children. This is
true not only in Africa, but in Asian and Latin American
cultures as well.

Why aren't condom distribution programs more effective?

Condom distribution systems are not always very efficient in developing countries, creating gaps in supply
and also exposing condoms to long periods of storage
and transportation in temperatures and other conditions that can damage them. Even at subsidized
prices, condoms can be too expensive for regular use
by the majority of people. (See p. 40.)

In a culture where impregnating a woman is enor-
mously valued, such as in Africa, men have not used
condoms, and women have rarely used birth control of
any kind. Men in developing countries find condoms
to be foreign to their experience.

Condoms are not popular in Asia or Eastern Europe,
even among those who are HIV infected.

Men in developing countries also lack access to

drug stores or other places where condoms are easily purchased. They often don't have places to store condoms where they will not be exposed to heat, sun and other elements. Condoms distributed in Africa are typically white latex, which feels foreign to African men. Many men feel condoms take away from the pleasure of sex.

Given these limitations, female condoms have been distributed more widely in Africa, providing women with the ability to provide their own protection during sex.

What are some of the other cultural factors affecting women?

In most developing countries of the world, women have few rights and choices in life. Many countries give them little legal protection, and most societies view them as being responsible for making their husbands happy, bearing children and caring for the family.

Countries that do have laws protecting women's rights have often managed to overcome male-dominated cultural beliefs and traditions. Where domestic violence against women is illegal, it is often not reported or prosecuted. Surveys done in some African countries reveal that both men and women believe that a husband has the right to beat his wife. Women have often reported being beaten for asking their husbands about extramarital sexual activity or for requesting them to use condoms.

FACT: Some countries have laws preventing women from owning property.

Women marry at very early ages and begin to have children as often as possible. A woman typically values having many children, both because of the high rate of child mortality and because having many children helps provide for the family and strengthen the family legacy. Women often have difficulties in childbearing since there are few doctors or medical facilities to offer help.

In situations where women are alone or girls are orphaned, it is easy for predators to force them into prostitution, enslave them as laborers or even force them to become child soldiers.

What are child soldiers?

Increasingly, rebel groups and others are either kidnapping children or attracting vulnerable children to become soldiers for their cause or provide sex for their soldiers. Child soldiers are defined by UNICEF as anyone under the age of eighteen who is part of a regular or irregular fighting force. It is impossible to estimate how many child soldiers there are worldwide, but there are tens of thousands. Girls who become child soldiers are often subjected to sexual violence and are vulnerable to becoming infected with STDs, including HIV.

Why do people believe so many myths about HIV in some countries?

Most people in developing countries have little formal education, no access to regular formal information such as the newspaper and no system of law that requires people to avoid making false claims. Given these realities, it begins to be more understandable that people would believe the myths about HIV, such as the belief that sex with a virgin can cure AIDS.

In the absence of formal health care, many poor people turn to traditional healers, who may be a cross between a doctor and a minister. Some are very good and promote practices that save lives and improve healing. Sociologists and anthropologists can point to many times when "educated minds" have dismissed claims of natural remedies only to eventually come back around to their effectiveness.

But traditional healers do not attend medical school and are not licensed. Some are very good and ethical, but others seek to control people and extract a livelihood from illnesses. Traditional healers have recommended many "cures" for HIV/AIDS because it is not in their interests to say the disease is incurable. Public health officials are now beginning to train some traditional healers so that they can incorporate sound medical advice into their traditional healing practices.

Just as people with fatal diseases in any country will try almost any type of medication or promise of a cure, so people in developing countries will naturally become more and more desperate as they see the people around

> "Health is what political leaders talk about if there's money left at the end of the day."
>
> Peter Piot, executive director, UNAIDS

them die. Fortunately, as more people are receiving treatment, they are able to dispel the myths and demonstrate the effects of proper medication.

Is it true that many people still believe in witchcraft?

Just as people in the United States might read their horoscope or follow the advice of a psychic, people of all religions sometimes rely on forms of witchcraft. Witch doctors are often happy to help spread rumors of supernatural forces so they can sell potions or remedies for combating it. But some so-called witch doctors are really closer to traditional healers, providing recipes to cure ailments.

Why would some people think AIDS is a plot launched by Americans?

Many Africans are grateful for the help provided by Americans. However, in many countries there is a history of fear and mistrust from the days of colonialism. At times, America has been viewed as exploiting certain countries for their natural resources or helping to bring about changes in leadership by encouraging coups. In 2001, Muammar Qadhafi, then president of Libya, charged that AIDS was created in a CIA laboratory.

President Thabo Mbeki of South Africa once claimed that there is no link between HIV and AIDS; he went so far as to appoint a health minister who promoted natural cures for HIV while warning of toxic side effects from ARTs.

Most of these leaders have now been replaced with those who understand the importance of obtaining treatment for their people, and who are working closely with the United States and other governments to bring health to their citizens.

Do people of certain religions have a lower incidence of AIDS?

Religion plays a role in the AIDS pandemic on many levels. Some religions encourage certain behaviors that seem to correlate to a lower rate of infection. Some religious leaders have been more involved in AIDS education than others. And some religions interpret their beliefs in ways that are more or less helpful to the spread of AIDS.

Some studies in Africa have shown that observant Muslims have a lower infection rate than other religions, even when measured in the same region. This is largely attributed to the fact that Muslim men tend to be circumcised—a practice proven to slow infection and transmission of the disease—while Christians and men following traditional religions tend not to be. But the difference may also be attributed to the fact that most Muslims live in West and North Africa, where the strain of HIV is con-

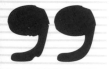

"[The AIDS crisis] is the greatest opportunity for the Church to be the Church."

Rick Warren, pastor, Saddleback Church

sidered less virulent, and that virginity is very important in the Muslim religion.

In addition, while many Muslim men practice polygamy, they tend not to have other partners besides their wives, so the chances of introducing the virus are lower than with men who have many casual partners.

While Christian churches have been promoting abstinence and faithfulness, so far no research has been able to indicate that church-going Christians have HIV/AIDS rates that differ from the general population. Christian churches have been at the forefront of caring for people with AIDS and organizing orphan care and support. But some experts believe that by hesitating to discuss sex and teaching early on that HIV infections only resulted from "sinful" behavior, Christians failed to be a more important factor in prevention.

Increasingly, leaders of all religions are speaking out about HIV/AIDS to promote responsible preventive behavior, encourage testing, reduce stigma, and mobilize care and support for those affected.

How is HIV/AIDS spread in different parts of the world?

In most countries, HIV/AIDS begins as a narrowly concentrated epidemic contained within "high-risk groups" such as intravenous drug users, prostitutes and homosexual men. Once the prevalence of infection reaches a certain level—about 1 percent—evidence suggests that the virus spreads rapidly to the general population through heterosexual activity.

The AIDS crisis in Eastern Europe and the former Soviet countries is primarily due to intravenous drug usage, especially among young people who are sexually active. Some reports say that heroin is now cheaper than alcohol, but needles are still expensive and are routinely reused.

Intravenous drug usage is also growing in China, where HIV infections were spread originally by unsafe blood-collection practices. Prostitutes spread the infection in some Asian countries, but Vietnam's infection rate was primarily attributed to intravenous drug usage.

In Latin America and the Caribbean, both intravenous drug usage and homosexual transmission account for most of the primary infections.

FACT: Brazil was the first developing country to implement a universal antiretroviral distribution program.

Is the rate of AIDS going up or down in developed countries?

There is great concern that HIV infections may be increasing again in wealthier countries. Education and media emphasis has waned, and people tend to think it is more of a problem for poor countries. And while the death rate has declined, since people who know they are infected have access to ARTs, the infection rate has remained steady. Public health officials estimate that as many as 18 percent of those who are living with HIV in the United States do not know they are infected. There is growing concern that "safe sex" is no longer practiced routinely, especially among young people.

What groups of people in developed countries are contracting HIV?

Sex between men (MSM; see p. 26) continues to be the most common way to be infected in the United States, Australia, Canada and several European countries. In the United States, urban areas showed the highest rate of new infections, and African Americans accounted for a disproportionate number of infections. In 2009, according to the Centers for Disease Control (CDC), Blacks accounted for 56 percent of AIDS-related deaths.

What are the Millennium Development Goals?

The Millennium Development Goals (MDG) were adopted by the UN in 2000 as goals that every country could hope to achieve by 2015. They are aimed at closing some of the gap between the "haves" and "have nots" of the world, and are meant to help poorer countries begin to set sound social policies. The United States as a country, and most humanitarian and religious groups in the developed world, support the MDG as basic rights and expectations for citizens of any country.

What is HPV? What does it have to do with HIV?

The human papilloma virus (HPV) is a virus common in almost anyone who is sexually active and is responsible for almost all cases of cervical cancer. HPV infections are more common and persistent in people living with HIV. Women living with HIV often have depressed immune systems, making them more susceptible to developing such diseases as cervical cancer.

Some countries have introduced HPV inoculations to girls before they become sexually active in order to prevent the virus from presenting. The Pink Ribbon Red Ribbon Initiative (www.PinkRibbonRedRibbon.com) encourages testing and treatment for HPV in poor countries, and also provides screening for breast cancer.

Millennium Development Goals

1. **Eradicate** extreme poverty and hunger.
2. **Achieve** universal primary education.
3. **Promote** gender equality and empower women.
4. **Reduce** child mortality.
5. **Improve** maternal health.
6. **Combat** HIV/AIDS, malaria, and other diseases.
7. **Ensure** environmental sustainability.
8. **Develop** a global partnership for development.

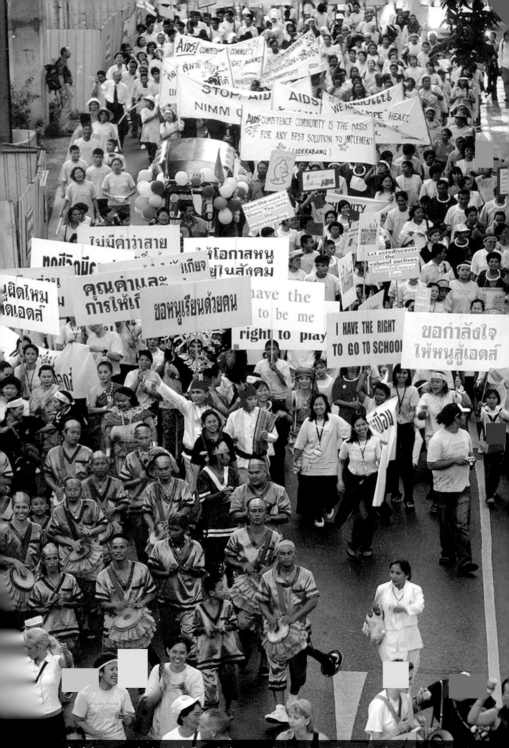

Activists march through Bangkok campaigning for safe sex and condom use

The politics of AIDS are as complex as the political systems around the world. So, too, are the laws concerning the disease.

Is it illegal to discriminate against people who are living with HIV or AIDS?

In the United States and other developed countries, for the most part, it is illegal to discriminate against anyone who is HIV-positive or has AIDS. Americans with AIDS are protected under some provisions of the Americans with Disabilities Act (ADA). Because it is now understood that HIV cannot be contracted through casual contact, children who are HIV-positive are less likely to be stigmatized by school systems. If their conditions are known, the issue is treated as confidential. Of course, this may not be how it works in practice, and American society must continue to fight this prejudice.

In many countries, people who are HIV-positive have ART covered by national health insurance. This has led some patients to move to countries where such treatment is provided free of charge. After the 2006 International AIDS Conference in Toronto, 160 people remained in Canada, seeking asylum because of their HIV status.

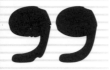

*"Stigma
remains the
single most
important
barrier to
public action.
. . . It helps
make AIDS the
silent killer."*

Ban Ki Moon,
secretary
general,
United Nations

However, people with HIV/AIDS in some parts of the world are not similarly protected. Many developing countries have no laws protecting people from discrimination. And even where laws exist, society continues to stigmatize those living with HIV. This contributes to a lack of interest in testing and means that many people remain in denial about their condition and may continue to infect others.

In some parts of the world, patients who appear to be HIV-positive are not welcomed in hospitals. Women who are HIV-positive may find it difficult to have their babies delivered in a hospital. In Eastern Europe and the former Soviet bloc countries, where HIV infections are spread primarily due to intravenous drug use, hospitals are struggling to develop appropriate procedures to deal with patients who are infected without further stigmatizing them.

Can a person who is HIV-positive immigrate to the United States?

Beginning in 1952, the United States restricted anyone from entering the country if "afflicted with any dangerous contagious disease." In 1987 Congress directed the US Department of Health and Human Services (HHS) to add HIV to its list of diseases of public health significance, drawing ongoing criticism from the international HIV/AIDS community for many years.

The United States Global Leadership Against HIV/ AIDS, Tuberculosis and Malaria Reauthorization Act of 2008 removed the statutory requirement that HIV be included on the list of diseases that barred entry in the United States. But the legislation did not change the existing regulations, and HHS continued to list HIV as a "communicable disease of public-health significance," requiring the more cumbersome visa process.

In 2009, President Obama signed an end to the ban, and in early 2010 HHS and the Centers for Disease Control and Prevention (CDC) removed HIV infection from the list of diseases that prevent non–US citizens from entering the country. Because of that, the International AIDS Conference was able to be held in the United States in 2012.

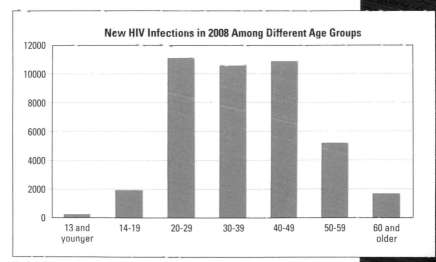

Estimated number of adults and children newly infected with HIV during 2008.

If I don't use IV drugs and am not sexually promiscuous, am I still vulnerable to infection?

FACT:
A severe shortage of health workers exists in many developing countries, potentially limiting treatment and testing facilities even if funding and drugs are available.

Public health officials agree that HIV infections are entirely preventable. While the disease is considered "communicable" because it can pass from one person to another, it is only contagious when a person engages in specific activities and comes in contact with the virus. The disease does not flow freely among a population. HIV cannot survive for long outside the body and is easily killed by sterilization.

The US blood supply is regularly tested, so the chance of infection from a transfusion is considered remote. Dentists and doctors sterilize their equipment, and disposable syringes have become the norm to prevent even accidental usage on more than one patient.

There are other public health risks associated with HIV, however, that may be more of a threat to the general population. People with depressed immune systems are easily infected with highly communicable diseases and may then become carriers of that disease. Tuberculosis, for example, is becoming far more common worldwide because those with suppressed immune systems acquire it more readily. Tuberculosis can become a major public health factor even for people who are not infected with HIV.

Why do some people advocate legalizing prostitution to help fight AIDS?

There is a growing debate internationally over whether it is better to recognize that the sex trade exists and therefore regulate and protect sex workers from becoming infected or spreading HIV infections. Some organizations feel that a person has the right to choose to become a sex worker. Other groups consider any transactional sex to be a fundamental violation of the dignity of a person and an immoral act.

Prostitution is already legal in many countries, including parts of Nevada in the United States. Some governments, such as Thailand, have continued to officially ban prostitution but have "unofficially" provided education, testing and protection about HIV to commercial sex workers (CSWs).

In some poor countries, children are enticed into the sex trade by being lured from the country to the city with promises of jobs. Because of the growing understanding that many prostitutes are infected with HIV, a higher price is paid for virgins in brothels. Sadly, this means that younger and younger children are being coerced or forced into prostitution. Although no one officially endorses such practices, those who favor legalization of prostitution sometimes argue that recognition and regulation of brothels would help eliminate the abuses of children. This is, of course, another controversial position.

"AIDS is becoming a chronic disease, requiring long-term solutions and sustained funding."

Paul Wolfowitz, former president, The World Bank

What is sex tourism?

People who travel from their own country to another country with the purpose of engaging in commercial sex are called sex tourists. Many are seeking young prostitutes, especially children, because they are believed to be less likely to be HIV-infected. Such activity is known as child sex tourism (CST). This practice is illegal in most countries, but it may not be enforced. Asian countries such as Thailand and Cambodia have been identified as destinations for sex tourists from the United States.

What is TIP?

TIP stands for Trafficking in Persons and is used most often in reference to an office in the US Department of State that tracks and tries to prevent the exploitation of people for sex, labor, slavery, servitude or organ removal. The US government strongly opposes legalized prostitution and believes that in countries where prostitution is legalized there is still a black market in illegal sex activity, often including trafficking victims. The TIP office has launched a campaign to educate Americans about the illegality of child sex tourism.

Why are women's legal rights limited in some developing countries?

Some countries have laws preventing women from owning property, voting and enjoying other rights we might consider basic. In some countries, women are banned from schools after a certain age; educational resources are limited, and boys are thought to deserve schooling more than girls. Marriage laws often allow girls to be married at a very young age, which further hurts their chances of pursuing an education or any form of independence. Other countries do not necessarily have laws that hurt women, but the practice of discrimination is widespread, and abused women have no recourse.

What are inheritance laws?

In some countries, women are not allowed to own land, so if a woman's husband dies, she is either thrown off the land, or the land passes to a relative of her husband's. She must marry him, become part of his family, or lose her land and possibly her children.

Because developing countries are often heavily agrarian, the land is an important family asset. When a father is designating his land for inheritance, he leaves the land only to his sons. But in some places, progressive fathers are beginning to leave land to their daughters as well.

Relatives may try to claim a widow's property after her husband dies, so one of the most effective ways to keep a woman from losing her savings is to give her a card which identifies her bank account by

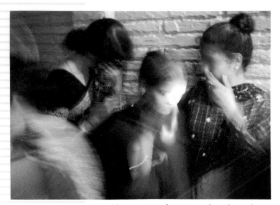

her fingerprint. This is being used in Malawi and has dramatically reduced the number of women who become destitute when their husbands die. Women in microfinance groups are also gaining access to insurance, which provides a small benefit for the burial of a family member and allows them to remain financially independent.

Young prostitutes anxiously wait as police raid their brothel in South Asia.

How important is it for country leaders to push for HIV testing and treatment?

Admitting that problems exist has never been a popular move for politicians or government leaders. While President Museveni of Uganda is widely praised now for his campaign against HIV/AIDS, in the early days of declaring war on the disease he created a great deal of discomfort in Ugandan society. Talk about sex was not common, and men did not feel they needed to be accountable for their sexual practices. Because of the openness about the problem in Uganda, many citizens found that they were stigmatized when traveling out of the country—in some cases even barred from entering certain countries.

Still, other countries have taken steps to curb the spread of infection or provide education, prevention and treatment. Senegal was one of the first countries to use a public campaign, enlisting Muslim clerics to help stop behaviors that might contribute to the spread of infection. Thailand's government became very aggressive about educating sex workers and promoting the use of condoms. Brazil has also been on the forefront of stopping the spread of HIV infections and providing free treatment to those infected.

An HIV/AIDS strategy is now part of almost every ministry of health program in the world. Access to assistance from the Global Fund and PEPFAR has helped many countries develop effective plans. But while the response to HIV/AIDS has helped create an infrastructure that can support other health initiatives, there is still less funding available for other diseases.

FACT:
HIV infection increases both the incidence and severity of clinical malaria in adults.

Is it true that Cuba has mandatory AIDS testing, and those who are infected are imprisoned?

Cuba was exposed relatively early to HIV/AIDS because soldiers from Uganda went there to train. In the early 1980s, Fidel Castro began to reject soldiers who carried a mysterious disease.

While Castro has been widely criticized for such practices as mandatory testing and other human rights violations, some have suggested that there may be something to learn from a country that suffers from widespread poverty but has managed to contain the HIV infection rate. In nearby Haiti, by contrast, the rate of infection has grown rapidly.

Many now suggest that the Cuban example may be helpful to other developing countries. Widespread education helps all Cubans understand how to prevent HIV/AIDS. Those who are HIV-positive are given access to free drugs and training on preventing transmission. The country is conducting extensive HIV/AIDS research. While those who test positive are placed in sanitariums, this is now done as part of a course of treatment and to help educate them on prevention methods.

Why is there so much discussion about international laws and agreements in regard to AIDS?

While each country must deal with HIV/AIDS by developing policies and enacting appropriate laws, the crisis is truly international and can only be effectively addressed on an international basis.

Human rights policies are largely driven by the UN. Trade agreements are subject to WTO policies. In many ways, the HIV/AIDS crisis forces nations to decide if they are willing and able to cooperate internationally.

What role does advocacy play?

Advocacy simply means to give a voice to a cause or to people who have no voice. In the United States, advocacy on behalf of AIDS was led early on by entertainers such as the late Elizabeth Taylor, who raised millions of dollars to help fight the disease and discrimination against those infected. Advocacy is primarily used to influence public opinion and policies. Singer Bono is one of the leading advocates on behalf of those affected by HIV/AIDS in Africa. Within church circles, Kay Warren of Saddleback Church, Lynne and Bill Hybels of Willow Creek Community Church, and others were early advocates on behalf of those living with HIV.

Many humanitarian organizations have led advocacy campaigns to increase funding for international HIV/AIDS prevention and treatment, and to bring attention to issues like orphans and violence against women.

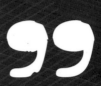

"*Every local church should be engaged in the war against AIDS.*"

Bill Hybels,
Willow Creek
Community
Church

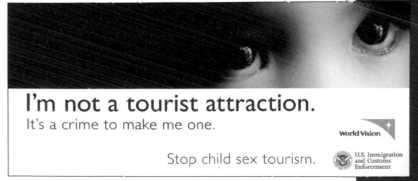

I'm not a tourist attraction.
It's a crime to make me one.

World Vision

Stop child sex tourism.

U.S. Immigration
and Customs
Enforcement

World Vision's program to combat child sex tourism uses billboards
such as this to deter abusers.

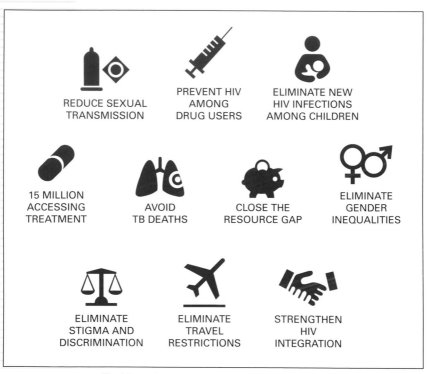

The UNAIDS 2011 Political Declaration: Targets and Elimination Commitments. Achieve universal access to HIV prevention, treatment, care and support by 2015.[5]

Are there broadly accepted prevention guidelines?

Individuals can reduce the risk of HIV infection by limiting exposure to risk factors. The World Health Organization has issued the following prevention guidelines.

1. Condom use. Correct and consistent use of male and female condoms can protect against the spread of sexually transmitted infections, including HIV. Evidence shows that male latex condoms have an 85 percent or greater protective effect against the sexual transmission of HIV and other sexually transmitted infections (STIs).

2. Testing and counselling for HIV and STIs. Testing for HIV and other STIs is strongly advised for all people exposed to any of the risk factors so that they can learn of their own infection status and access necessary prevention and treatment services without delay.

3. Pre-exposure prophylaxis (PrEP) for HIV-negative partner. Antiretroviral drugs taken by the HIV-negative partner can be effective in preventing acquisition from the HIV-positive partner, depending on risk level and other factors.

4. Post-exposure prophylaxis for HIV (PEP). Post-exposure prophylaxis (PEP) is the use of ARV drugs within 72 hours of exposure to HIV in order to prevent infection. PEP is often recommended for health care workers following needle stick injuries in the workplace.

5. Male circumcision. Male circumcision, when safely provided by well-trained health professionals, reduces the risk of heterosexually acquired HIV infection in men by approximately 60 percent.

6. Elimination of mother-to-child transmission of HIV (eMTCT). The transmission of HIV from an

99

"Being involved with AIDS care has revived the name of the church."

Cyprien Nkiriyumwami, church relations director, World Relief Rwanda

HIV-positive mother to her child during pregnancy, labor, delivery or breastfeeding is called mother-to-child transmission (MTCT). MTCT can be fully prevented if both the mother and the child are provided with antiretroviral drugs throughout the stages when infection could occur.

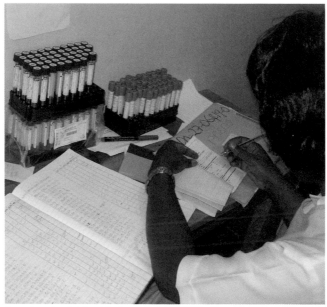

A nurse records blood test results from HIV testing.

FACT:
About 40,000 new HIV infections occur each year in the United States.

7. *ART.* A new trial has confirmed that if an HIV-positive person adheres to an effective antiretroviral therapy regimen, the risk of transmitting the virus to their uninfected sexual partner can be reduced by 96 percent. For couples in which one partner is HIV-positive and the other HIV-negative, WHO recommends ART for the HIV-positive partner regardless of her/his immune status.

8. Harm reduction for injecting drug users. People who inject drugs can take precautions against becoming infected with HIV by using sterile injecting equipment, including needles and syringes, for each injection.[6]

"

"Our church members now know how to welcome a person with AIDS into the church as a human being."

Juvenal Ngedahaya, Association des Eglise Inkuru Nziza, Kigali, Rwanda

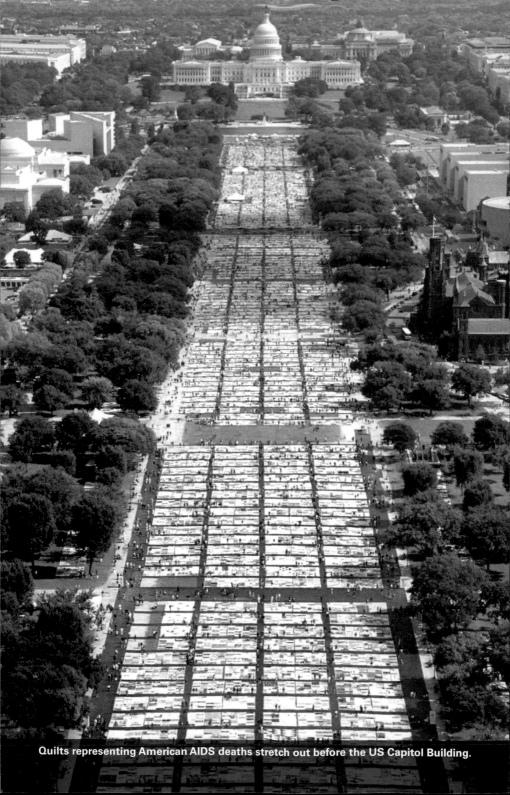

Quilts representing American AIDS deaths stretch out before the US Capitol Building.

Learning the facts about the AIDS pandemic is the first step. But how can anyone really make a difference? Here are some thoughts.

What can one person do that will change the situation?

There's a saying in Uganda: "One plus one soon makes a bundle." When Ugandans were dealing with an HIV infection rate that threatened to wipe out a considerable portion of their population, they learned the importance of each person doing something to change the situation. So, too, each of us can dedicate ourselves to doing something to make a difference.

The first thing we can do is become educated. Reading this book is part of doing that. Sharing it with someone else is another step. Reading the books listed in the bibliography or visiting the websites listed are also important steps.

You can also receive daily updates from the Kaiser Health Network (www.kff.org), which does an excellent job of covering all aspects of HIV/AIDS.

Writing to your member of Congress, Senator or other public officials to encourage funding for AIDS issues is an important step toward making sure that those in public office understand that their constituents care about the pandemic.

Funding is crucial to prevent and treat HIV/AIDS. Giving to a charity involved in AIDS, even if it's only a small gift, is an important step to take.

How can I get my congregation involved?

Congregations, service clubs, schools and other groups all have the potential to raise awareness and significant funds for fighting HIV/AIDS. Studies have shown that when faith leaders and congregations become involved in educating and caring for those with HIV/AIDS, they are able to reach people missed by other programs. In addition, providing a safe place for those living with HIV or engaging in risky behavior to seek counseling and treatment is a key component to prevention and lowering infection rates.

You might start by forming a task force or offering a class on HIV/AIDS. There are materials available from denominations as well from the ONE campaign (www .ONE.org). You could hold a fundraiser for HIV/AIDS research and bring a speaker in to talk about the situation.

Saddleback Church in California has provided many resources to congregations wanting to get involved in a ministry to those with HIV/AIDS. Go to the website www .purposedriven.com and click on the HIV/AIDS section.

You can order some of the free materials available from UNAIDS, WHO, the CDC and many other humanitarian organizations, and place them in your church or school library. (More resources are listed at the back of this book.)

How do I decide which charity to support?

You might start by deciding if there is some area of the crisis that is especially of interest to you. Are you interested in educating people about HIV and helping prevent its spread? Do you feel a special desire to help AIDS orphans? Do you feel an affinity toward a particular country?

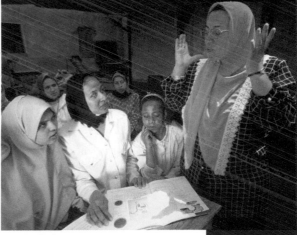

Some organizations are especially involved in prevention, while others deal primarily with treatment. Some are focused on the needs of women, and some work exclusively with children.

Some organizations spend much of their time advocating for causes related to AIDS such as legal rights for women. Some are dedicated to making drug treatments available for a wide number of people.

A women's group receives health training in Egypt.

Many faith-based organizations are involved in various aspects of HIV/AIDS work, so you might want to support an organization that is consistent with your background and upholds your beliefs. You might also check to see if your denomination or faith has a related medical mission.

Will I be able to get involved directly?

There are many opportunities to get involved with fundraising, administrative work and AIDS education in the United States. But opportunities to go overseas are generally limited to people with some medical training or other relevant professional background.

Individuals with nursing degrees and medical training are needed to work in developing countries. Doctors Without Borders is one of the most well-known organizations sending medical staff overseas, but there are a variety of medical missions looking for individuals.

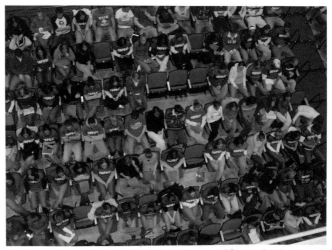

Student activists with World Vision's Acting on AIDS wear "orphan" T-shirts representing children who are orphaned by HIV/AIDS in Africa.

What major should I pursue in college to get involved in HIV/AIDS issues?

Almost any major can prepare you for working on some aspect of the HIV/AIDS pandemic. Mathematicians are needed to analyze statistics and issue reports. Journalists are needed to tell the stories of those dealing with HIV/AIDS. Teachers will be needed to continue educating children and adults about the pandemic. While the greatest need is in health care, researchers are also needed to study treatment options.

Many humanitarian organizations employ people with backgrounds in economics, education, sociology, psychology and other fields, depending on where they are working. You can go to www.interaction.org to see the types of organizations involved in this aspect of humanitarian work and what the prerequisites are for jobs. Then you can go to the website of each organization and see what types of jobs are available. Jobs are also posted on www.reliefweb.int, www.Idealist.org or www.philanthropy.com.

You may want to pursue a graduate degree in public health, international development, education or psychology, depending on your particular interest. It is also helpful to become fluent in a second language. If possible, try to work as an intern in an international humanitarian organization to begin to understand what area particularly interests you.

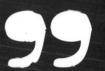

"This is the time to show that the church is not a mausoleum for saints, but a place of hope for the sick."

Rev. Christo Greyling, World Vision

How do I know what data to trust?

Most organizations consider UNAIDS and WHO as the official sources of information (that is why they are used for most of the data in this book). You can go to the websites at www.unaids.org or www.who.org to find statistics, free publications and much more information. For US statistics, the CDC is the best source (www.cdc.gov). The National Institutes of Health also has information (www.nih.gov).

How can I help people in my community who are HIV-infected?

Local organizations working with HIV-infected individuals often need volunteers to do everything from delivering meals to helping patients pick up their prescriptions, to assisting with fundraising or answering the help line. Call a local HIV/AIDS organization in your community or find out if your faith community has an outreach to those with HIV. Or contact your local Red Cross or Salvation Army, or go to www.charitynavigator.org to find a list of charities working in the area. Starting in our own communities is an important way to reach out. If you find that no group is working in your area, find out what the needs are and see what you can do.

Acknowledgments

This book is really the result of the efforts of many people. Research for the first edition was done by Kate Wilkinson and Chase Bourke. It was edited by Angela Lewis and reviewed by Ann Claxton and Patton Dodd.

For this edition, John Kraemer offered invaluable updates and reviews. Kay Warren, in addition to her tireless and ongoing efforts, was willing to write a foreword during a particularly busy time in her life.

This edition was designed by Beth Hagenberg, edited by David Zimmerman and laid out by Jeanna Wiggins.

Many humanitarian groups contributed quotes, photos, publications and data to this book as part of their ongoing commitment to the cause of HIV/AIDS. We hope the entire book offers a resource for them to use in their work.

Finally, thanks to all those who have been working on this cause for a very long time and whose tireless efforts have done so much to move us forward in understanding and compassion. May this be one more contribution to the much larger effort.

Selected Bibliography

30 Years into the AIDS Epidemic. UNAIDS, 2011.

100 Questions & Answers About HIV and AIDS. Joel Gallant. Jones and Bartlett Learning, 2012.

2012 Report on the Global AIDS Epidemic. UNAIDS, 2012.

African Development Indicators—2012. World Bank Africa Database. The World Bank, 2012.

The AIDS Dictionary. Sarah Barbara Watstein. Facts on File, 1998.

AIDS in the Twenty-First Century. Tony Barnett and Alan Whiteside. Palgrave, 2002.

The AIDS Pandemic. Lawrence O. Gostin. University of North Carolina Press, 2004.

The AWAKE Project. Compiled by Jenny Eaton and Kate Etue. W Publishing, 2002.

Black Death. Susan Hunter. Palgrave, 2003.

Breaking the Conspiracy of Silence. Donald E. Messer. Fortress Press, 2004.

Global AIDS: Myths and Facts. Alexander Irwin, Joyce Millen and Dorothy Fallows. South End Press, 2003.

HIV/AIDS—The Faith Community Responds. Pamela Potter, editor. Georgetown University Press, 2004.

HIV/AIDS in Africa. Ezekiel Kalipeni, Susan Craddock, Joseph R. Oppong and Jayati Ghosh, editors. Blackwell, 2004.

HIV/AIDS Prevention and Education. Ken Casey, executive editor. World Vision, 2003.

HIV/AIDS Surveillance Report. Public Health Service, CDC. Department of Health and Human Services, 2012.

The Invisible People. Greg Behrman. Free Press, 2004.

The Lazarus Effect. Lance Bangs, director. RED, 2010.

Moving Mountains: The Race to Treat Global AIDS. Anne-Christine D'Adesky. Verso, 2004.

The No-Nonsense Guide to HIV/AIDS. Shereen Usdin. Verso, 2003.

Religion and AIDS in Africa. Jenny Trinitapoli and Alexander Weinfeb. Oxford University Press, 2012.

Rethinking AIDS Prevention. Edward C. Green. Praeger, 2003.

Trafficking in Persons Report. Staff of US Department of State, Office to Monitor and Combat Trafficking in Persons. US Department of State Publications, 2012.

"Who Is AIDS?" Kate Wilkinson. University of Connecticut Dissertation, 2004.

The World Health Report 2012. World Health Organization, 2012.

Diagrams and photographs in this book are provided by the author, with the following exceptions.

p. 30: Pharmaceutical worker in Bangkok. Photograph by Reuters.

p. 38: HIV and AIDS education program for young people. Photograph by UNAIDS/O. O'Hanlon.

p. 44: An NGO-led HIV and AIDS information session. Photograph by WHO/UNAIDS.

p. 45: HIV-positive man sitting at home. Photo by UNAIDS/O. O'Hanlon.

p. 49: Estimated adult and child deaths from AIDS during 2010. Diagram by UNAIDS/WHO.

p. 52: An illustration showing where antiretrovirals block HIV. Diagram by NAM, www.aidsmap.com. Used by permission.

p. 64: Adults and children estimated to be living with HIV in 2010. Diagram by UNAIDS/WHO.

p. 66: Talekelini Kagaso displays her "smart card." Photograph by Opportunity International.

p. 71: Top six government donors to the Global Fund. Data taken from *The Global Fund 2010 Annual Report*.

p. 90: Activists march through Bangkok. Photograph by Reuters.

p. 93: New HIV infections in 2008. Graph produced by Hans Villarica/MEDILL.

p. 98: Young prostitutes anxious wait as police raid their brothel. Photograph by Ted Haddock/International Justice Mission.

p. 101: World Vision's program to combat child sex tourism. Copyright ©2004 by World Vision. All rights reserved.

p. 102: The UNAIDS 2011 Political Declaration. Icons by UNAIDS.

p. 106: Quilts representing American AIDS deaths. Photograph by Reuters.

p. 109: A women's group receives health training. Photograph by UNAIDS/G. Pirozzi.

p. 110: Student activists with World Vision's Acting on AIDS. Photograph by World Vision.

Recommended Websites

www.AIDS.gov
US government site for resources on HIV/AIDS.

www.AIDSMap.com
UK website for those living with HIV/AIDS.

www.AVERT.org
UK-based international AIDS charity.

www.theBody.com
Comprehensive guide to the best info on HIV/AIDS.

www.CARE.org
Website of nonprofit active in HIV/AIDS work.

www.CDC.gov
Website of the Centers for Disease Control and Prevention.

www.TheGlobalFund.org
The international fund to fight tuberculosis, malaria and AIDS.

www.joinred.com
Website for a campaign fighting for an AIDS-free generation.

www.KaiserNetwork.org
The Kaiser Family Foundation's portal to AIDS information.

www.NIH.gov
The National Institutes of Health home page.

www.ONE.org
A campaign against extreme poverty and diseases including AIDS.

www.PurposeDriven.com
The source of HIV/AIDS information for churches.

www.UNAIDS.org
Statistics and other resources on the global pandemic.

www.UNICEF.org
Information on children and their global struggle.

www.USAID.org
Website of the US Agency for International Development.

www.WHO.org
The World Health Organization's website.

www.WorldBank.org
Organization dedicated to fighting global poverty.

www.WorldVision.org
Largest faith-based organization working on AIDS.

Notes

[1] The "State-Sponsored Homophobia" report from the International Lesbian, Gay, Bisexual, Trans and Intersex Association (ILGA) lists seventy-eight countries and five other political entities with laws against homosexuality. Accessed October 29, 2012, at http://old.ilga.org/Statehomophobia/ILGA_State_Sponsored_Homophobia_2012.pdf.

[2] World Health Organization press release, May 30, 2007, accessed October 29, 2012, at www.who.int/mediacentre/news/releases/2007/pr24/en/index.html.

[3] Jill McGivering, "Aids Takes Deadly Toll in China," *BBC News*, February 18, 2009.

[4] For more information on Saddleback Church's support of orphan care in Africa, visit www.orphansandthechurch.com.

[5] UNAIDS, 2011 Political Declaration: Targets and elimination commitments. Accessed October 30, 2012, at www.unaids.org/en/targetsandcommitments/.

[6] WHO Fact Sheet Number 360, July 2012, HIV/AIDS.

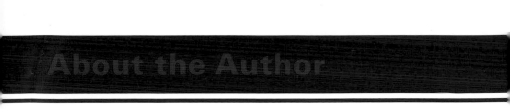

About the Author

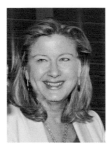

Dale Hanson Bourke is president of PDI, a marketing and communications strategy firm. The author of ten books and numerous magazine articles, she often speaks and writes on international development and women's issues. Previously president of the CIDRZ Foundation and SVP at World Relief, Bourke has also served as publisher of Religion News Service and editor of *Today's Christian Woman*, and was a nationally syndicated columnist.

A graduate of Wheaton College, Dale holds an MBA from the University of Maryland and has served on the boards of World Vision US, World Vision International, International Justice Mission, Sojourners, ECFA and Opportunity International. She currently serves on the board of MAP International and the Center for Interfaith Action on Global Poverty (CIFA).

www.DaleHansonBourke.com
Twitter: @DaleHBourke
Facebook: facebook.com/SkepticsGuides

Do you wish you understood some of the most complicated issues of our times? Would you like help navigating these sometimes divisive subjects? Then the Skeptic's Guide™ series is for you. Each book answers the most often asked questions, illustrating concepts with photos and charts, and even showing different points of view.

The Israeli-Palestinian Conflict sheds light on the places, terms, history and current issues shaping this important region, providing a framework for Christians to use in understanding why the conflict occurred, why it continues—and what remains to be done.

In *Immigration,* a heavily debated topic is broken down into easy-to-understand facts, charts, quotes and answers. The book is a great primer for anyone who wants to understand why immigration has become such a controversial topic.

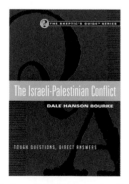

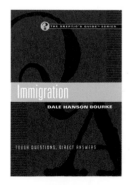

The Israeli-Palestinian Conflict	*Immigration*
(available now)	(available spring 2014)

www.ivpress.com/skepticsguides